62
NATURAL WAYS
TO BEAT
JET LAG

CHARLES B. INLANDER & CYNTHIA K. MORAN

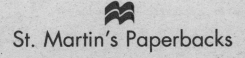

St. Martin's Paperbacks

62 NATURAL WAYS TO BEAT JET LAG

ISBN: 0-312-96325-4

Printed in the United States of America

St. Martin's Paperbacks edition/November 1997

10 9 8 7 6 5 4 3 2 1

THE AIR TRAVELER'S TOOLBOX:

eyedrops
wraparound dark glasses
earplugs
sugarless chewing gum and candy
lumbar pillow
moisturizer
saline spray
toiletries
travel alarm
DO NOT DISTURB sign
slippers
bottled water

LEARN TO DESIGN YOUR OWN
CUSTOM TRAVEL KIT WITH

62 NATURAL WAYS
TO BEAT JET LAG

Contents

62

NATURAL WAYS
TO BEAT

JET LAG

CHAPTER 1

Understanding Jet Lag

It's 5:30 A.M. in London. You've just exited the jetway of the 6:00 P.M. flight from New York. You feel as though you've been wearing your clothes for a week, and you could swear your shoes have shrunk two sizes.

Your mouth and nose are dry, your head is pounding, and your eyes sting. Your stomach feels twice its normal size, as though it's filled with cement. Forget food: you'd settle for a swallow of antacid liquid. A minute ago you were sweating; now you feel cold. You're so tired that nothing makes sense except a ten-minute nap on the bench next to the luggage carousel.

You feel terrible—what's going on?

Flu? Onset of a dread disease? Nope. Just jet lag. Jet lag occurs when your body's rhythms are out of synchronization with the clock time at your destination. In short, jet lag occurs any time you travel east or west and abruptly cross two or more time zones. Jet lag is the temporary desynchronization that occurs between the time you land and the time when all of your body's systems adjust to the time change.

But take heart. This unpleasant, disorienting condition is a temporary state, and there are many preventive measures you can take before you even step onto the plane, as well as preventive *and* therapeutic ministrations for the time you're actually in the air and after you land.

What Causes It?

Jet lag is not affected by the distance you fly. What *does* make a difference, however, is whether you are flying across the earth's meridians (east or west) or in line with the earth's axis (north or south). If you cross no time zones on a north-south flight—from New York to Ecuador, for instance— even though you are flying a long distance, you will not experience jet lag. Why? Because you have not crossed a time zone.

According to Richard Dawood, M.D., writing in the April 1994 *Condé Nast Traveler,* the intensity of your jet lag is determined by the *minimum* number of time zones between you and your destination. For instance, you'll cross fifteen time zones flying an easterly route from the East Coast to Sydney, Australia, but only nine if you fly west to get there. Jet lag intensity will be based on nine.

Before we talk more about jet lag, though, it will help to review some fundamentals of sleep, because the sleep-wake cycle is at the center (and bears the brunt) of jet lag's desynchronizing effects.

Internal Clocks

The human body is governed by two complex timing devices: one to promote sleep (the circadian clock), the other to promote awakening (the homeostatic clock). (The homeostatic clock is also known as the "buildup and decay clock." It is reset daily by hormones and hormonelike brain chemicals called *neurotransmitters* as they are used up during the day and replenished at night.) Together they constitute our circadian (from the Latin *circa* meaning "around" and *dian* meaning "day") rhythm, the 24-hour human cycle of "about a day."

The homeostatic clock runs on a slightly longer schedule than the circadian clock. Thus, for normal sleep, synchronization of the two timekeepers is critical. Scientists explain that we achieve this daily coordination and maintain our body's rhythms by responding to time cues called *zeitgebers*. Zeitgebers may be external: social cues, such as the dinner hour, clock time, work, or exercise;

or environmental cues, such as dark and daylight. Zeitgebers may be internal, such as the digestion of food or medication, or the brain's release of melatonin to signal sleep.

While a person's natural circadian rhythm can range anywhere from twenty-two to twenty-eight hours, most adults' bodies run on a twenty-five-hour clock. As a civilization, we have forced the twenty-five hours into a tidier twenty-four-hour rhythm that matches the sun's twenty-four-hour daylight and dark pattern as the earth rotates east to west. Tuned to this cycle of light and darkness, the human brain's circadian timing mechanism permits people throughout the world to live on reasonably synchronized daily schedules.

A key function of the circadian clock is to control body temperature, the strongest internal cue in the sleep-wake cycle. When our temperature is highest, we are most alert and function the best. When it is lowest, we are most ready for sleep or rest. For most adults, the two high-temperature times in the twenty-four-hour cycle happen in midmorning and again in midevening. The two temperature "troughs" occur five to seven hours after the highs—at between 2 P.M. and 5 P.M. and again sometime between 3 A.M. and 5 A.M. It's at these times that we are most tired and our judgment and physical coordination are at their worst. It's a bad time to run a marathon or make an important business decision. Clearly, then, the time you schedule that important meeting in London is critical. (We'll have more to say about this in chapter 2.)

When daylight occurs at a different time from a traveler's home time zone, the circadian clock—cued by the daily light-dark cycle—goes askew. (Indeed, jet lag is technically known as *circadian dysrhythmia,* or circadian rhythm disorder.) Your body is not sure whether to stay on its established internal schedule, the pull that is the strongest, or to follow light, and dark, and environmental cues at the new destination. It starts following strong external zeitgebers almost right away, switching over entirely once your body adjusts to the new time zone and emerges from jet lag.

What Are the Symptoms of Jet Lag?

They're many and varied. "Initially, on the first day at your destination," notes jet lag specialist and author Charles F. Ehret, Ph.D., in *Overcoming Jet Lag,* "you begin to notice that you have an ever-growing sense of exhaustion that is far more pronounced than the general fatigue with which you left the airplane. It is an all-over, all-consuming weariness that affects your sense of time and place and well-being, as well as your concentration, memory, and performance."[1] In fact, studies show that jet lag can decrease your physical ability and mental acuity by up to 20 percent.

[1] New York: Berkley Publishing, 1983.

When jet travel discombobulates our circadian clock, we throw more than one hundred bodily functions or systems into temporary disarray.

Notable Times of Day

- Peak alertness times: 9 A.M.–noon; 7 P.M.– 10 P.M.
- Alertness troughs: 3 A.M.–5 A.M., 3 P.M.–5 P.M.
- Peak physical powers: early evening
- Least sleepy time: 6 P.M.–9 P.M.
- Best time to nap: 2 P.M.–4 P.M.
- Best time for simple, repetitive tasks: late afternoon
- Best time for short-term memory tasks: early morning
- Best time for logical reasoning: midday
- Least sensitivity to pain: early morning

Adapted from *Esquire,* October 1994, p. 127.

Some Human Cycles Disturbed by Jet Lag

Rapid (Ultradian)	*Daily (Circadian)*	*Weekly / Monthly (Intradian)*

Heart
  heartbeat
  pulse rate
	Heart
	  blood pressure
	  blood clotting
		Reproduction
		  ovulation
		  menstruation
		  hormone levels

Rapid (Ultradian)	Daily (Circadian)	Weekly / Monthly (Intradian)
Lungs breathing perspiration	Eyesight visual acuity	
Cell division	Mental ability alertness cognitive function memory depth perception judgment reaction time	
Eye blinking	Physical ability physical prowess energy levels rest-activity sense of pain	
Swallowing	Sleep-wake	
Brain waves	Digestion bowel movements urinary output hunger pangs Reproduction hormone levels Temperature Metabolism Sense of time Hair growth beard	

Adapted from *Overcoming Jet Lag*, by Charles F. Ehret, Ph.D., and Lynne Waller Scanlon (New York: Berkley Books, 1983), p. 21; and *How to Sleep Like a Baby*, by Dianne Hales (New York: Ballantine Books, 1987), p. 124.

Other early symptoms are likely to include disorientation, confusion, off-schedule bowel and urinary movements, hunger at the wrong times, and even some memory loss. The gastrointestinal system pumps digestive acid and enzymes into the stomach when there's no food to digest. New light and dark times upset production schedules of neurotransmitters, which govern, among other things, our ability to fall and/or stay asleep. Normal cellular waste removal and replenishment become temporarily chaotic, resulting in diarrhea, constipation, abdominal cramps, or sometimes all three in sequence.

Later symptoms, says Ehret in *Overcoming Jet Lag,* may consist of lack of sexual interest, limited peripheral vision, decreased muscle tone, impaired night vision, reduced physical work capacity, disrupted phases of body rhythms and functions, slowed response to visual stimulation, reduced motor coordination and reflex time, insomnia, acute fatigue, loss of appetite, and headache. The impact of prescription drugs may be altered, too.

Research suggests that it takes the body twenty-four hours per time zone crossed to fully readjust. On a trip from the United States to the Orient, for instance, in which you cross some twelve time zones, it will take nearly two weeks to fully and completely acclimate after you land. However, it is equally true that there are natural ways to prevent and treat many of jet lag's manifestations.

Who Gets Jet Lag?

No human being is exempt from jet lag, and that means passengers as well as pilots, new flyers, and frequent flyers.

Indeed, human beings are not the only cyclical beings. Other animals follow circadian patterns, but they don't usually get jet lag (unless they are being transported by plane across time zones).

On their own, most animals can't travel east or west with the speed of airborne humans. And east-west migratory patterns of various faster-traveling animals and birds, such as Canada geese, show an innate instinct of resting a few days at each stop, limiting their east-west flights, and traveling more in northerly or southerly directions.

A variety of factors can affect jet lag's intensity in different people.

East versus West Travel

To fly across time zones in a westerly direction—to an earlier time of day—lengthens the traveler's day, while to fly east—where it is later in the day—shortens it. Studies show that without time cues, or zeitgebers (which range from alarm clocks to regular, self-imposed wakeups, meals, bedtimes, and presleep rituals) to make us function on a twenty-four-hour schedule, most of us would probably run on a twenty-five-hour clock. Thus the human tendency toward a longer day makes jet travel to the west—called *phase delaying*—an easier adjustment than flying east.

This is especially true for "night owls," people who are most alert after 10 P.M. For these travelers, flying west creates less discomfort because it may seem just like another day of staying up late. While flying east, or *phase advancing,* may be somewhat easier for "larks," those who naturally rise easily in early morning hours, easterly jet travel tends to pack more of a jet lag punch for everyone, since humans do not adapt as well to a shortened day, one that is "less" than twenty-four hours.

Age

At various stages of our lives, our circadian rhythms change, running longer or shorter than the twenty-four-hour circadian pattern. Adolescents, for instance, run on a longer schedule (slower clock) of about twenty-seven hours. (An adolescent's internal clock says it's only 9 P.M. when it's really midnight.) Older people run on a shorter rhythm (faster clock) than twenty-four hours, with many awakening for the day well before 6 A.M. These circadian rhythm changes make people, as they age, more vulnerable to missing their deepest, or most restorative, sleep during travel. And fatigue always exacerbates jet lag.

Timing

The time of arrival—a result of flight schedules that put the flyer into his or her destination literally in the middle of the night or very early morning, according to point-of-origin time—is an external cue that foretells the severity of jet lag.

In upcoming chapters, we talk more about how these variables can affect your vulnerability to jet lag and what you can do to lessen, if not eliminate, their effects on your mind and body.

Which Team Will Win?

Jet lag can be a special nemesis for athletic teams playing a transmeridian game schedule. Research shows that if their home fields are on the West Coast or in Hawaii, traveling east across two or more time zones to play a day game can be a killer.

In one of the first studies published on the subject of jet lag and athletic teams, twenty-seven National Football League teams' performances were reviewed by researchers who analyzed nine years (1978–1987) of win-loss records and compared them to time zone and game time changes. When games were played within the same time zone, researchers determined, the home team enjoyed a home field advantage, leaving the visitors only 43.8 percent chance of winning.

When traveling to play eastern rivals, even allowing more than a day and a half (forty-two hours) ahead of game time to acclimate, the visiting West Coast teams lost increasingly more of an edge as they moved east, with only a 35.9 percent chance of winning against a central time zone rival and a 33.7 percent chance of winning in an East Coast competition. When a western team flew to the East Coast even earlier (forty-eight hours in advance) and advanced their practices (and, thus, time adjustments) by three to four hours to match East Coast scheduling, their odds of beating the home team increased by 2.3 to 46.1 percent.

Notably, a subset of this research involved some teams' participation in anti–jet lag adjustments, which appeared to eliminate the downturn in performance.

Night games told a different story. In the same time zone, night games showed a 76.3 percent home field advantage, an average that remained consistent whether the West Coast team played rivals from the same time zone or were visited by central or eastern time zone teams for night games. The western teams continued to hold the winning advantage in night games in central or eastern time zones.

The studies underscore that eastbound travel (moving game times to earlier in the day) is consistently a more difficult adjustment and results in lower performance for teams crossing more than one time zone without employing any anti–jet lag measures. Why are western teams favored in night games? First, a home team always has the advantage of playing on its own field, whether teamed against local or eastern cross-continental rivals. Then, for western teams visiting central or eastern time zone competitors and playing a night game, game time is closer to their regular West Coast schedules.

A University of Massachusetts study of nineteen North American Major League baseball teams based on the East and West Coasts reported results similar to the football findings. Those teams traveling from east to west, the easier adjustment, scored more runs and won more than those traveling in the opposite direction.

The studies make several important points for teams traveling east with an intent to win: they must either a) fly to the game destination far enough ahead of time to fully adjust to the new time zone, probably at least two full days ahead for West Coast teams playing in the East, or b) start pretrip, anti–jet lag adjustments employing a combination of natural measures.

While baseball and football teams have been the subjects of the primary studies cited, transmeridian travel affects any competitive athletic event. For this reason, serious athletes plan their cross-country travel painstakingly, choosing not only the time of day they arrive at a destination, but also how many days in advance of the meet, game, or competition they should fly for best results.

The Influences of Food, Light, and Activity

Research points increasingly to food, light, and activity as the strongest influences on resetting the biological clock—they are deeply interrelated. The food we eat affects production of brain chemicals—neurotransmitters—that signal particular body rhythms to turn on or off. One such rhythm is the sleep-wake cycle, governed also by our exposure to bright light. When light enters the eye, the amount of serotonin metabolized into melatonin—both neurotransmitters that relax and prepare us for rest and sleep—is curtailed, which begins the waking process. As the body cycles toward waking, other neurotransmitters—epinephrine, norepinephrine, cortisol—are secreted and initiate the activity phase of the rest-activity cycle. Research indicates that activity may be almost as important a cue to the body's clocks as light.

Discovering the Switchpoint

In their early research on how light exposure affects the activity of melatonin (the brain chemical that effects sleep), pioneer chronobiologists Alfred J. Lewy, M.D., Ph.D., and Thomas A. Wehr, M.D., discovered the *phase-response curve* (*PRC*), the predictable correlation in humans between the time they are exposed to light and the timing of their circadian rhythms.

Subsequent research has found that a person's circadian rhythms are delayed by light exposure early in the evening. Sitting in bright light at dinnertime, for instance, turns your clock back to an earlier time, just as though you were flying west. But light exposure very late at night or in the very early morning has the opposite effect and, instead, advances the body's rhythms. To be in bright light at 11 P.M. or 2 A.M. makes your body clock go forward—and feel as though it is later than it actually is, as though you were flying east. Researchers call the median point, where light exposure stops delaying and begins advancing the circadian rhythms, the *switchpoint*. Studies have determined that the switchpoint in the majority of adults occurs at around 4 A.M. (slightly later for night owls and slightly earlier for larks).[2]

Light exposure a few hours *before* the switchpoint causes the most pronounced rhythm delays, while light exposure *after* the switchpoint prompts the most intense advances. Understanding the switchpoint and its relationship to phase-delaying and phase-advancing circadian rhythms is the fo-

[2]Oren, Dan A., M.D., et al. *How to Beat Jet Lag* (New York: Henry Holt, 1993).

cal point of light therapy for fighting jet lag (see Chapter 2).

The Neurotransmitters That Affect Jet Lag

Let's take a closer look at these brain chemicals. Scientists now know that the manufacture, release, and use of at least six neurotransmitters—cortisol, epinephrine, norepinephrine, dopamine, melatonin, and serotonin—figure prominently in the sleep-wake cycle and circadian rhythms. Here's a quick primer on them:

• **Cortisol** (also called hydrocortisone) controls metabolism and emotions and stimulates the body's recovery from stress. Cortisol supply in the body peaks at 6 A.M. and runs down about midnight. When it runs into short supply at day's end (as it is naturally supposed to), the action cues body temperature to fall and the mind to wind down, become less alert, and prepare for sleep. Drowsiness results.

• **Epinephrine** (adrenaline), **norepinephrine** (noradrenaline), and **dopamine** are the neurotransmitters most active during periods of stress, emergency, or alertness. They enliven the brain and make you more attentive, motivated, and mentally energetic. Tyrosine, an amino acid found in many protein foods, is the precursor used to produce these brain chemicals. To manufacture these brain chemicals, the nervous system uses *precursors,* components that it finds in the body's naturally occurring amino acids or breaks down from amino acids gained from protein food sources.

• The ebb and flow of **melatonin** helps cue sleep-wake cycle rhythms. Melatonin secretions are stimulated by darkness; indeed, studies show we have ten times more in our systems at night than in daytime. The minute that daylight (or almost any light, according to new research) intrudes, melatonin production shuts down until the next scheduled sleep cycle (or the arrival of darkness).

• **Serotonin,** manufactured from the amino acid tryptophan by the hypothalamus gland, is believed to control states of consciousness as well as mood and sensitivity to pain. Like cortisol, it is thought to affect body temperature changes and, thereby, the sleep-wake cycle. Scientists believe serotonin accrues in the body during deep sleep. With its calming, sedative effects, serotonin release is especially useful in treating anxiety-related disorders, and some doctors use serotonin-producing drugs to treat jet lag. Tryptophan, the amino acid that occurs naturally in our bodies as well as in many protein foods, is a precursor of serotonin, and studies indicate that serotonin is a precursor of melatonin. (See chapter 5 to find out more regarding melatonin.)

Jet Lag and the Latest Research

Much of the current chronobiological research has centered on how light cues the brain—and thus the circadian clock. Only recently have scientists established that along with activity and rest, light and dark are *the major zeitgebers* that set our biological rhythms and that our eyes play key roles interpreting in the light-dark function. Studies show that our retinas are networked by nerve connectors to two tiny nerve groups called the suprachiasmic nuclei (*SCN*), located behind the eye in the brain's hypothalamus gland. The SCN have naturally occurring electrical rhythms that react to light and dark impulses sent from the retina and thereby initiate the resetting of our internal clocks.

SCN nerves connect to other nerves in the hypothalamus using those chemical messengers called neurotransmitters. This partnership starts and stops a variety of physiological processes. One such function is to the pineal gland at the base of the brain. Through this partnership SCN stimuli initiate nighttime secretion of melatonin (the sleep-inducing neurotransmitter) in the pineal gland.

The Biggest Breakthrough

For decades, scientists and medical practitioners have labored to develop a cure for jet lag. In the natural arena, various diets that depend on timing and prescribed types of food have been recommended, while other approaches have advocated use of herbals and natural supplements, special exercise programs, different sleep schedules, and even meditation. Each of these can claim partial success, but none—including drug therapy—has yet proved to eliminate jet lag.

At the end of each of the next three chapters, anti–jet lag therapies using food, light, and action are suggested. These particular tips are set off from others because they are a) the most vital for beating jet lag, b) inextricably linked, and c) dependent on precise application, sequencing, and timing. Our regular text suggests supporting tips: Unlike food, light, and activity therapies, they needn't all be done, nor do they need to be carried out in any particular order.

Melatonin therapy—an extension of light therapy—is excluded from these special sections, appearing instead in chapter 5, "The Promise of Research." Many travelers take synthetic melatonin capsules and report excellent results in cutting jet lag's duration. In fact, controlled, limited studies indicate that synthetic melatonin may be one of our greatest "natural" sleeping pills. However, because melatonin is a natural substance, it falls outside the domain of any regulatory agency and currently reaches the public principally through health food stores, supermarkets, and drugstores. Even though synthetic melatonin counts many research scientists and medical doctors among its supporters, until it is reclassified as a drug or otherwise regulated, users cannot be sure of the pills' purity or strength. In the interim, if you follow the information provided in the special boxes in chapters 2 through 4, you'll find they lead to results remarkably similar to those of melatonin therapy.

Jet lag can be worsened or helped by what you choose to do before, during, and after your flight. While light therapy is likely to have the biggest impact on reducing jet lag's effects, using a combination of the other complementary tips will give your light therapy an added boost in helping to vanquish the condition that every long-distance flyer dreads.

CHAPTER 2

What to Know Before You Go

You now know that jet lag is a temporary physiological disorder that affects every human being who abruptly flies across two or more time zones. Fortunately research has provided a variety of approaches for beating jet lag's most debilitating effects. You *can* succeed in minimizing jet lag by using a combination of natural tips, beginning with your pretrip planning and activity.

If you're a leisure flyer with advance time to put your trip together thoughtfully, you'll be traveling at an advantage and able to employ a number of these suggestions. If you're a frequent time zone—crossing flyer, we've noted tips we think have special application to frequent flyers. Whatever kind of traveler you are, mix and match to find the combination that works best for you.

There are four areas to consider in the final months, weeks, and days prior to your departure: planning and scheduling; health and fitness; diet and nutrition; and packing and logistics. Each area has a distinct reason for attention, and if any or all are ignored or delayed until just before departure, the result is unnecessary stress. Stress takes a mental and physical toll, ultimately diminishing your immune response and making you susceptible to colds, flu, and other illnesses. If your body is in the fight-or-flight mode—the classic stress response—it has fewer reserves to devote to overcoming jet lag, lengthening the time it takes you to recover from your trip. Pretrip planning will help you eliminate last-minute stress, and smooth the way for a more comfortable arrival at your destination.

Advance Work: Two Weeks to Several Months Before Your Trip

Planning and Scheduling

1. Add yourself into the jet lag equation.
Consider the personal variables we've already mentioned (age and your sleep-wake rhythms) and place them in the context of your trip (travel direction and arrival time). Consider such other

personal factors as how well rested and stress-free you will be at trip time and if you're in peak health or on the comeback from an illness. Since your mind can deeply affect how your body reacts, consider if you have an upbeat attitude about where you're going and if you're open and flexible to the change associated with different surroundings and schedules.

It will also help if you have an understanding of how long the worst symptoms of untreated jet lag are likely to last on your trip.

Calculating Jet Lag

The conventional wisdom recommends from one-half to one full day of recovery for every time zone crossed. Thus a traveler flying from Chicago to Paris—a seven-hour time difference—could expect to feel normal after several days to a week (even though some less noticeable bodily systems might still be adjusting).

But what if companies can't afford such luxurious R&R time? How can they determine the *absolute minimum rest time* they should schedule for employees who need to recoup the necessary mental acuity to conduct or participate in an important meeting or business undertaking? Canada's Civil Aviation Organization came up with the answer, according to Donald Kowet, author of *The Jet*

Lag Book, with its "Jet Lag Resynchronization Formula."[1] To work the formula, you need to know the following:

- total hours travel time (time in air plus on the ground, if flight is not nonstop)
- the U.S. time zone from which you'll be traveling
- departure and arrival times of your flight (in local times)
- how many time zones you'll be crossing? (Don't forget to factor in daylight savings time for your time zone, if it applies, and ask your travel agent if your destination country follows daylight savings, too.)
- the following "coefficient" table:

Departure Period	*Departure-Time Coefficient*	*Arrival-Time Coefficient*
8 A.M. to Noon	0	4
Noon to 7 P.M.	1	2
7 P.M. to 10 P.M.	3	0
10 P.M. to 1 A.M.	4	1
1 A.M. to 8 A.M.	3	3

[1]New York: Crown Publishers, 1983.

Then plug the numbers into the following formula:

[Travel time (in hours) divided by 2] +
[Number of time zones in excess of 4] +
[Departure-time coefficient] +
[Arrival time coefficient] = Rest period (in tenths of days)
Divide this figure by 10 =
Number of days rest needed (rounded up to the next figure).

[*Source:* Kowet, Donald. *The Jet Lag Book*. New York: Crown Publishers, 1983.]

It's easier than it looks. Here are illustrations:

Example 1: An eastbound flight from **Chicago to Paris**, leaving at 5 P.M. (CT) and arriving at 8 A.M. (Paris time), crossing seven time zones, involving eight hours of travel time: [8/2] + 3 + 1 + 3 = 11/10 = 1.11 (two days rest).

Example 2: A nonstop westbound flight from **San Francisco to Hong Kong**, leaving at 2 P.M. (PT) and arriving at 7 P.M. the next day (Hong Kong time), crossing sixteen times zones, involving thirteen hours of travel time: [13/2] + 12 + 1 + 2 = 21.5/10 = 2.15 (three days rest).

Example 3: An eastbound flight from **New York to Bangkok with a stop in London**, leaving at 9 P.M. (ET) and arriving in London 9 A.M. (London time), crossing five time zones, involving seven hours of travel time; three hours layover; leaving London noon (London time) and arriving in Bangkok 6 A.M. the next day (Thailand time), crossing seven time zones, involving eleven hours of travel time. Trip total: twelve times zone crossed, with a total travel time of twenty-one hours. [21/2] + 8 + 3 + 3 = 24.5/10 = 2.45 (three days rest).

Example 4: A westbound nonstop flight from **Philadelphia to Los Angeles**, leaving 2 P.M. (ET) and arriving 5 P.M. (PT), crossing three time zones, involving six hours of travel time. [6/2] + 0 + 1 + 2 = 6/10 = .6 day (one day rest).

Remember: The length of recuperative time is also influenced by the times of day you depart and arrive, as well as your own personal factors.

═══════════════════════════════

2. Try to schedule nonstop flights whenever possible, unless you're on a trip of more than six hours' flight time.

On longer trips, if your schedule permits, you can help alleviate some of jet lag's punch with a one-day or longer stopover along the way (often at no or little additional cost). A stopover can help your mind and muscles stay more limber, while assisting your body clock with a more gradual time change adjustment than it would have if flying all at once. For instance, flyers who travel from New York to Sydney, Australia, crossing nine time zones on a direct flight that stops briefly in Los Angeles, takes twenty-one hours. If schedules permit, they may elect a two-day stay in Los Angeles, resuming their trip forty-eight hours later.

By turning one marathon trip into two shorter

ones, the flyer has two days to fully acclimate to the first time shift before making the final adjustment to the last times zones crossed.

3. Be selective about aircraft.

Larger aircraft usually are less cramped, with more room to walk, stretch, even spread out for sleeping, and often offer passengers more spacious seating arrangements. Boeing 747s, 777s, and 767s, DC-10s, L-1011s, and Airbus 320s are large planes that tend to be more passenger-friendly than Boeing 727s and 737s, and DC-8s. So-called wide-body planes, such as the 747, generally seat nine across in more generous space than other planes, like the 737s, which often seat two passengers on one side of the aisle, three on the other.

The airline or your travel agent can tell you what plane flies where. Since seating configurations differ by airline even on the same model plane, ask to see the airline's seating chart when you're making your choice.

4. Choose your seat in advance, and be selective.

Seating that allows for maximum mental and physical comfort is important to helping prevent jet lag. Request a seating assignment and boarding pass at the time of your reservation.

A midplane seat closest to the wing affords the most stable ride, seats in the rear of the plane the least. Seats just behind the emergency doors and bulkheads (walls of the cabin) allow the most leg room, yet each has disadvantages. These disadvantages (armrest tray tables and no underseat stowage) may be worthwhile trade-offs to you. Emergency door row seating has special requirements (no children or physically challenged people), and bulkheads are usually where parents traveling with infants are seated. In most planes several rows of seats have restricted reclining range, which is detrimental to the traveler on long flights, where changing sitting position and resting or sleeping are vital to fighting jet lag. They include the last row of most cabins (except in first class) and the row immediately in front of emergency exits.

On long flights—when you are crossing more than two time zones and sleep or rest is important—try to avoid seats near areas of high activity: the galley and the lavatories. Further, calculate when you'll be sleeping and choose a seat on the opposite side of the plane from where the sun will be shining when you are trying to sleep.

Consider, too, these other seating issues: An aisle seat gives you more leg room but may mean you have to get up more often—possibly during sleep times—when inner seatmates want out. A window seat, while more cramped, is a better sleeping seat because there is less disturbance by restless seatmates.

Also, before departure, check if any center section seats are open. Often two or three seats are available together. Take one and spread out over the empty ones upon departure.

5. Control your arrival time, if possible.

On flights longer than two hours, jet lag will affect your sleep schedule—the farther you travel, the more the disruption. Therefore it's best to find a flight that will get you to your destination *as close to your normal bedtime in the new time zone as possible*. These examples demonstrate the importance of smart booking:

Eastbound: When booking a seven-hour flight from New York to London—a five-hour time difference—if your normal bedtime is 10 P.M. (ET), look for a flight that leaves close to noon to get you to your destination by 7 P.M. ET (midnight London time). Then you'll be able to go directly to bed upon arrival at your hotel. If, on the other hand, you take a 6 P.M. flight from New York (the time a majority of transoceanic flights depart), you'll be arriving at 1 A.M. ET but 6 A.M. London time. That's another fourteen hours until bedtime. *Remember:* The later in the day you fly east, the longer your day will be before your new 10 P.M. or 11 P.M. bedtime.

Westbound: If you are taking the six-hour flight from New York to San Francisco (a three-hour time difference), booking an evening flight (8 P.M. ET) will get you to your destination at

11 P.M. PT, allowing you to go to sleep as soon as you get to your hotel. (It'll be 2 A.M. home time, still only a couple of hours out of sync with your normal bedtime.) *Remember:* The earlier in the day you fly west, the longer your day will be before your new 10 P.M. or 11 P.M. bedtime. (East=fly early. West=fly late.)

6. Don't schedule meetings or sight-seeing tours too soon after you arrive.

Studies suggest that jet lag diminishes mental and physical performance by as much as 20 percent—a significant factor if you want to be at your business best or in your most enthusiastic tourist mode shortly after you arrive. If you have the final word in arranging your ground schedule, try to allow at least a night's sleep, preferably a whole day's rest, before doing strenuous mental or physical activity. If that's out of the question, schedule activities at times when your destination city is "open for business" that also coincide with the time period when you would normally be most alert. Using the New York–London example, set your business meeting between 12 noon London time (7 A.M. New York time) and London's close of business at 5 P.M. (noon New York time).

Health and Fitness

7. Lighten up.

Without even trying, you're going to feel heavier during jet travel because of two physiological changes that occur in a pressurized cabin. First, at cruising altitude, your cabin will be pressurized to between 5,000 (equivalent to the air in Denver) and 7,500 feet (equivalent to air in Mexico City), pretty thin air for those of us accustomed to living closer to sea level. With less air pressure, there is a natural tendency toward swelling as body gases expand, making your stomach feel full, fat, and bloated. Second, when you sit for long periods of time, gravity pulls body fluids to the extremities, making your feet, legs, and hands swell—and with less air pressure, they swell more than usual. Some flyers can "gain" as much as four pounds from edema in their legs during a long flight, according to an April 1994 *Condé Nast Traveler* article.

Once you factor in the ever-shrinking size of a coach-class airplane space (equal to confinement in a twenty-by-thirty-two-inch box for several hours) and the relatively small size of airplane seats (varying from eighteen to twenty inches wide by twenty-nine to thirty-four inches front to back in economy class), you should be convinced that staying as trim as possible when you travel will pay off in comfort (and health) dividends.

You don't need to go on a pretrip crash diet. Just follow these health-promoting tips in the time leading up to travel:

- *Eat healthfully and observe regular mealtimes.*
- *Avoid high-fat, high-carbohydrate, processed foods.*
- *Cut out empty calories* by moderating your intake of (or avoiding) alcohol, sugary soft drinks, and candy.
- *Drink fluids copiously,* at least eight 8-oz. glasses of water or low-sugar juices daily, to maintain cellular health and bodily waste removal.
- *Exercise.* If you're doing regular exercise to maintain your best weight, you'll also breathe more easily in the plane's thinner air; help maintain sound mental health by releasing endorphins, brain chemicals that give you a sense of well-being—a positive attitude and low stress translate to fewer and shorter debilitating effects of jet lag; boost your immune system, improving your resistance to germs encountered in the plane's close quarters; and improve muscle tone and strengthen bones, aiding in preventing your limbs, back, neck, and joints from becoming too stiff (and prone to injury) from long periods of sitting during your flight.

8. Leave stress at home.

As we've noted, stress worsens jet lag. When you're a victim of long-term stress, you're living in a fight-or-flight stance, with all of your hormones, muscles, blood cells, and energy reserves directed to fighting off the "attacking" problem. This means fewer bodily resources are available to help you over the jet lag hump. Review and identify what areas of your life are most stressful a few weeks in advance of your trip:

- *Work on finishing what you can and delegating what you don't have time for* if it's work that's at the root of your stress. If you find it stressful to be out of touch, arrange a few set times when you'll check in by phone, answering machine, or fax—and don't deviate from the schedule.

- *Try to deal with the most intense stressors on the home front before you go.* If a duty or chore can't be deferred until your return, perhaps another member of the family can take on the responsibility.

- *Learn deep-breathing exercises before you go.* These are geared to making you inhale and exhale to the fullest—bringing a higher volume of oxygen into your body than when you are doing shallow, worried breathing—thereby helping expel cellular waste from your body. Deep-breathing exercises will also help you in-flight, especially if you are a white-knuckle flyer.

9. Guard your health.

A challenged immune system is an open door to greater jet lag symptoms. For this reason, it's paramount that your immune system be at its strongest when you fly. It's not just airline lore that germs circulate on planes. Whenever many people are in such close proximity for as long as a transmeridian flight, the odds of being exposed to a cold, flu, or other contagious illness increase. Moreover, airplane air is dry and recirculated, and even though it's supposed to be filtered before recirculation, it is not the same as breathing freely outdoors or even indoors, where there is likely to be more space.

In the days preceding a trip, give extra thought to commonsense precautions and behavior that will help you resist colds, flu, and other contagious illnesses. Remember:

- *Wash your hands regularly and often.* This is the most surefire way to avoid transporting germs into your body. Always try to use an antibacterial soap (the label will so indicate).
- *Avoid touching your nose, eyes, and mouth.* These "cavities" are the doorways through which cold and flu germs pass into your system.
- *Avoid situations where many people congregate* or small children are present, and defer visits to sick friends or family. These are prime areas for picking up viruses or illness-causing bacteria. If you don't avoid these gatherings, wash your hands immediately upon leaving.

- *Get adequate sleep*—good advice always, but especially apt in the time leading up to a trip, a period when you may feel the need to skimp on rest in order to pack and attend to the many other details involved in getting out of town. Sleep-deprived people lack top mental acuity and are not in peak condition to fight jet lag. (We have more to say about timing your sleep schedule in this and subsequent chapters.)

- *Practice good home hygiene.* Don't use others' towels, pillows, face cloths, and so on, all of which can harbor cold germs. Use an antibacterial soap; wipe down phones, light switches, and other commonly touched objects; and regularly empty wastebaskets containing used facial tissues (and then wash your hands).

- *Get a flu shot and take other medical precautions* if you are vulnerable to certain conditions—for example, get a pneumonococcal vaccine to prevent pneumonia recurrences, especially if you are in a high-risk category (over sixty, prone to respiratory diseases, living or working in an indoor setting where many people congregate, suffering from any cardiovascular, pulmonary, or other organ-weakening disorder or disease, or are around small children, who are natural germ carriers).

10. Take care of sinus problems and allergies.

The human ear is a mechanism highly vulnerable to damage as airplane pressure changes (a time when the pressure against the inside of the eardrum must readjust to the new pressure against the outside of the eardrum). If your nose or ears are clogged during takeoff or landing—perhaps you're among the one in five adults who suffer from seasonal allergies or someone who experiences occasional and/or chronic sinus congestion—the equalization activity by the body is compromised. Permanent ear damage can result.

- *Be alert to the signs of a developing sinus infection, and see your doctor* if you have one. You'll know by a nasal discharge that's turned from clear to yellow or green and by the tender areas just above the bridge of the nose or below the eyes accompanied by a persistent headache. The longer a sinus infection is left to fester, the more difficult it can be to eliminate, so act quickly.
- *If you suffer from allergic rhinitis* (congested nasal passages from exposure to allergens), *be sure to take the antihistamine or decongestant* your doctor recommends, to keep your condition from leading to a sinus infection.

11. Get flight clearance from your doctor, if you've been ill.

Here are a few preflight medical recommendations from Eden Graber and Paula M. Siegel in their *Traveler's Medical Companion:*[2]

[2]New York: William Morrow, 1990.

- After surgery, *leave adequate recuperative time* (at least ten days to three weeks after head or heart surgery, and then fly only with your doctor's approval).
- If you have a flare-up of a chronic gastrointestinal disorder such as colitis or diverticulitis, *have the condition treated and in remission before you fly.* (They suggest waiting for three weeks, until after the symptoms leave and you receive a medical go-ahead.)
- *If you are exposed to or come down with a contagious disease*—strep throat, measles, chicken pox, German measles, whooping cough—decide with your doctor when it will be safe (to you and others) to travel again.

Common sense dictates that air travel is not sensible if you are still sick, especially if you are still contagious. Your immune system may still be fighting the germ and not prepared or strong enough to fight off the additional germs you may pick up on the plane or from jet lag. Finally, traveling when you are still able to spread a disease—whether it's a cold (some types of cold are contagious for a week or two after you've first shown symptoms) or the flu, strep throat, or chicken pox—is inconsiderate to others, especially to those who may have compromised immune systems or are pregnant.

If you're worried about losses you'll incur if you need to reschedule or if you feel it's likely that an illness—recurring or new—will insert itself in your travel picture, you may want to consider purchasing trip insurance that covers just such an instance. Check the travel section in your library or bookstore or on the Internet for details.

12. Learn to relax on command.

Tension and anxiety, whether from a fear of flying or problems you are facing connected with your trip, are bad stressors that will have negative consequences on the length and intensity of your jet lag. Relaxation exercises are a proven way to combat stress because they eliminate stressful thoughts and defuse your stress response. The objective is to invoke concentration on command that allows you to clear your mind of everyday, external thoughts while you focus inward, on your senses. Achieving the relaxation response triggers the release of endorphins, those "feel good" neural chemicals we've already mentioned.

Many different relaxation exercises exist. Here are three easy classics, which can be modified for use in-flight, too:

- **deep breathing:** Close your eyes and sit or lie in a comfortable position. Pull shoulders back as you inhale deeply, letting air fill you, starting with your diaphragm and progressing to your chest cavity. Hold for three seconds. Exhale, letting shoulders drop. Repeat until you feel less tense.
- **progressive muscle relaxation:** Close your

eyes and, as you sit or lie in a relaxed position, start at your feet and visualize one group of muscles at a time, relaxing each along the way. Continue until you have progressed through your entire body, and/or feel the tension depart and a feeling of weightlessness set in.

- **meditation:** The classic consciousness-altering exercise that allows you to clear your mind and heighten your awareness of involuntary body rhythms (breathing, heart rate). Find a comfortable seat, or lie down, then close your eyes. Select a special, one-syllable word (your mantra) and repeat it to yourself continuously. If your mind wanders, direct it back by concentrating on your mantra. Continue for twenty minutes, at which time your entire body and mental state should be relaxed and tension-free.

Diet and Nutrition

13. Eat nutritiously.

Admittedly, before a trip even the best-laid plans can go awry as you race to finish undone projects and last-minute details. It is without doubt a time, however, when you need to pay extra attention to what you eat. By avoiding foods with "empty" calories (those that do not add nutrients, but do add body fat) and eating nutritiously in the week or two preceding a long trip, you will fortify your immune system and energy reserves. This will keep you in fit shape on the plane and help you throw off the effects of jet lag more quickly once you arrive. Foods can give you long-lasting energy and alertness (proteins), instant energy that quickly dissipates into sleepiness and energy reserves when eaten in moderation (carbohydrates), or extra weight and indigestion if eaten in excess (fats).

14. Put vitamins and minerals in your life.

Vitamins are the thirteen organic substances required to regulate the functioning of cells, and minerals are the thirteen-plus chemical elements that must be present in the diet to maintain good health. According to the U.S. Department of Agriculture, however, at least a third of Americans consume less than 70 percent of the Recommended Dietary Allowances (RDAs) of vitamins A and C, the B-complex vitamins, and the minerals calcium, iron, magnesium, and zinc.

Here's a quick look at the RDAs for these immune-boosting, antioxidant vitamins and minerals. Remember, though, the RDAs were created to establish the *minimum* amount of a vitamin or mineral needed to avoid a deficiency; hence RDAs typically are at low dosages. (RDAs, in parentheses, are for twenty-five- to fifty-year-old men and women.)

Vitamin A: essential to immune-system stimulation and production of the substance that lines the respiratory tract. A deficiency weakens these membranes. Beta-carotene, a vitamin A derivative, helps increase disease-fighting T-cells. Without vitamin A, cilia "slough" off and cells lose their ability to secrete mucus; consequently, cold or flu viruses and other germs entering the nasal passages are not trapped and expelled. Mucus also contains lysozyme, an enzyme that destroys microbes, including viruses. (women: 8,000 IU; men: 10,000 IU).

Vitamin C: boosts immunity against colds and other infections, combats heart disease, helps prevent cancer, and speeds up wound healing. It is essential to the manufacture of connective tissue, which is found throughout the body, and helps maintain tissue structure. Like vitamin E and beta-carotene, vitamin C also acts as an antioxidant. Antioxidants are substances that roam the body, bonding with and neutralizing harmful molecular fragments called free radicals. Antioxidants also help neutralize potentially harmful reactions in the body. (women and men: 60 mg daily; smokers: 100 mg)

The B complex vitamins:

- **thiamin** (B_1): helps cells convert carbohydrates into energy. (women: 1.0–1.1 mg; men: 1.2–1.5 mg)
- **riboflavin** (B_2): helps cells convert carbohydrates into energy and is essential for red

blood cell growth. (women: 1.2–1.3 mg; men: 1.4–1.7 mg)

- **niacin** (B_3): aids in the release of energy from foods and helps maintain healthy skin. (13–19 mg)
- **pantothenic acid**: vital for food metabolism and the production of essential body chemicals; helps adrenal function and antibody formation. (no RDA available; experts recommend 4–7 mg/day)
- **pyridoxine** (B_6): aids in chemical reactions of proteins and amino acids and in forming red blood cells. (women: 1.6 mg; men: 2.0 mg)
- **biotin**: expedites the metabolism of protein, carbohydrates, and fat. (no RDA available; experts recommend 30–100 mcg/day)
- **B_{12}**: central to red blood cell production (2 mcg/day)

Other important vitamins in your diet include antioxidants D, which helps maintain blood levels of calcium and phosphorus (5 mcg or 200 IU/day), and E, which helps form red blood cells and may improve immune function in older people (women: 8 mg; men: 10 mg).

Folic acid: important in normal cell growth and protein metabolism; deficiency weakens the immune response. (women: 180 mcg; men: 200 mcg)

The Health-Promoting Minerals Include:

- **The mineral calcium:** Building of bones and teeth is calcium's most familiar role. Calcium is also essential for nerve conduction, muscle contraction, heartbeat, blood clotting, the production of energy, and the maintenance of immune function, among other things.

- **The mineral iron**: A deficiency in this mineral causes immune dysfunctions, including shrinking of lymphatic tissue, defective functioning of several disease-fighting substances, and fewer fighter T-cells. (women: 10–18 mg; men: 10 mg)
- **The mineral zinc**: Zinc is critical to the immune system because it helps initiate antibody production and is active in the circulation of disease-fighting T-cells. (women: 12 mg; men: 15 mg)

If you're eating regular, nutritious meals, you may be getting the full RDA of many of these vitamins and minerals in your food. If not, often just adding a good multivitamin to your daily regimen will be all that it takes. Megadosing is not recommended and may even be harmful to your health. Check with your medical practitioner before starting a new vitamin and mineral regimen.

15. Eat on a regular schedule.
You already know that exposure to light is the most important environmental cue that signals your sleep-wake clock. But did you know that eating meals on a regular schedule is one of the most important *social* cues? You see, the digestive system receives its signal to prepare for the arrival

of food from internal cues sent by brain chemicals, and from the body's acclimatization to your regular eating schedule.

At mealtimes, the digestive system releases into your stomach the natural acids that will help break down foods. If food is not forthcoming, you wind up with an upset stomach. Conversely, if you consume a pizza at 3 A.M., your digestive system is thrown off-guard, with none of its functions primed to accept food, especially any containing fats, which are the most difficult to digest. The body then must initiate an emergency digestive response that uses more energy and draws blood and activity away from other body processes, disrupting their schedules. The result can be waking at wrong times (or outright insomnia) and indigestion or heartburn, as the body tries to cope with its off-schedule burden.

Jet lag places extra strain on this complex system by requiring it to phase advance or phase delay to accommodate your new destination time (see Chapter 1). If your system is already in disarray because of irregular mealtimes, you are apt to find that jet lag will hit you harder and longer.

16. Drink plenty of fluids.

Airplanes are notorious for their dry, desertlike air, which easily dehydrates you. (The relative humidity inside the cabin is only 2 to 10 percent—normal is 50 to 60 percent.) Dehydration intensifies jet lag's effects because it prevents cells from being properly nourished, cleansed of toxins, and replenished. This in turn results in the body working at suboptimal levels. Recent studies have shown that a majority of American adults are regularly dehydrated and don't even know it. (If you're thirsty, experts agree that you're probably already 30 percent dehydrated.)

Vital to the proper functioning of every organ, water flushes your system, washing out cellular toxins as it rehydrates you. In the course of a normal day, the body depletes roughly eight cups of liquid just on normal body processes such as sweating, urination, and digestion. That's why doctors recommend that you regularly drink at least eight 8-oz. glasses of water or juice a day. (Make sure you're not counting coffee, caffeinated sodas, or alcoholic drinks, whose diuretic qualities dehydrate you further.) You can also add to your body's fluid balance by consuming high-water-content items such as vegetables and fruits. If you're wondering how much water is enough, follow the advice one doctor gives to his patients: Observe the color of your urine. If it's pale, versus a deep yellow, you're probably drinking enough fluids.

17. Cut down on your caffeine and alcohol, and if you smoke, stop.

All three habits have negative effects on your sleep, and since sleep deprivation is a major player in poor jet lag adjustment, you should eliminate from your pretrip schedule any sleep disrupters. Too much caffeine makes you anxious and can delay sleep onset, while alcohol and smoking generally allow you to get to sleep but interrupt your sleep cycle by waking you with rebound effects in the middle of the night.

These three substances are stressful to your body in other ways as well. Studies show, for instance, that stress-related hormones are higher in coffee drinkers (or tea drinkers, chocolate eaters, and those who drink caffeinated sodas). As we've already noted, caffeine and alcohol are diuretics that dehydrate you. For every ounce of alcohol you drink, more than an ounce of fluid is removed from your body, while essential infection-fighting vitamins (A, B, and C) are also depleted. So taper down on both before you fly (the exception is when following jet lag specialist Charles Ehret's anti–jet lag diet, which calls for expunging coffee and other xanthine-containing foods from your diet within three days of travel, then ingesting the same substances at particular intervals during travel to advance or delay your body's clocks).

A Word about Diet

One of the original anti–jet lag diets—published in 1983 in his book *Overcoming Jet Lag* and still widely followed—was devised by Charles F. Ehret, Ph.D., of Argonne Laboratories in Illinois. The diet's efficacy, however, is a matter of some contention. Some travelers find it highly effective; others are skeptical. Studies do show, however, that Ehret's work is valid as a jet lag minimizer. Research on food/brain interactions and other anti–jet lag food strategies support his two main tenets concerning eating:

- The body clock resets quicker when glycogen (the body's main stored energy) is depleted in the liver. (His diet achieves this by alternating feast and fast days preceding travel.)
- Xanthines, a class of chemicals that include caffeine, are effective tools for delaying or advancing the biological clock.

Our suggestions for fighting jet lag with food also cite the work of Judith Wurtman, Ph.D., author of *Managing Your Mind and Mood through Food*.[3] The MIT neurobiologist has researched the effects of food on the mind and body for more than thirty years. You may choose to follow Ehret's very specific anti–jet lag diet reviewed here or incorporate the more general recommendations of Wurtman and others. Either way, disciplining yourself to follow the correct diet is imperative to your success at beating jet lag.

Smoking dries out the nasal passages, a first line of defense in filtering out germs—and one of

[3]New York: Harper & Row, 1986.

the first parts of the body, along with the eyes, to be irritated by the dry air in the airplane. Research shows, too, that smokers are more prone to respiratory diseases and infections. If you're a smoker, airline regulations require you to abstain from smoking on all U.S. domestic flights and on 80 percent of all flights from the United States to foreign destinations. So if you're in the habit, start breaking it before you board.

Plot your anti–jet lag strategy

It will be easiest to make calculations if you set a second watch, called your travel watch. In this example, we'll consider the normal bedtime 11 P.M. and waking time 6 A.M.; daytime = 6 A.M. TO 6 P.M.; nighttime = 6 P.M. to 6 A.M.

Eastbound timing: Each day you will advance an hour—set your watch one hour later—until you "catch up" to destination time (DT). From the East Coast to London is a difference of five time zones. The ideal anti–jet lag light strategy calls for you to begin your pre-trip strategy five days before arriving at your destination. Five days before your trip, set your travel watch one hour ahead of HT (home time), the second day two hours ahead, etc., until you have "advanced" your travel clock to DT, London time.

Westbound timing: Each day you will set your clock back one hour per time zone until you "back up" to your DT.

Eastbound light: Get brightest light in the very early morning. Since you will be waking an hour earlier each day in your home time zone—6 A.M. on your travel watch—you may need to seek bright light from artificial sources from waking time through sunrise. Once the sun is up, try to get outdoor light if feasible for another hour or so. Try not to wear sunglasses, but, to protect your eyes, don't stare directly at the sun, either. Following our example, you will want to avoid bright light any time after mid-afternoon. If it's still daylight in HT when you are going to bed at 11 P.M. on travel time, you'll want to wear your mask. Avoid brightly lit places such as malls after mid-afternoon on your travel time; if you must be near bright lights, wear dark glasses.

Westbound light: Avoid bright light in the morning, since you want your body to feel as though sunrise is later. If you get a few days' headstart on your anti–jet lag program, it means you will probably need to wear a mask until waking time— 6 A.M. on your travel watch. Wear sunglasses through midday, then extend "daylight" into late afternoon, using artificial light, if need be.

The Final Countdown: Just Before You Leave

Our overview begins within the week before you travel. For longer flights, especially those heading east, consider adapting your schedule beginning three to five days before you leave, if feasible. Conversely, those traveling only two zones east or west needn't begin more than a day before travel.

Start by setting your travel watch to destination time (DT).

Pretrip Light Strategies

The original light therapy schedule for advancing or delaying body clocks was developed by circadian researchers Alfred J. Lewy, M.D., Ph.D., and Surge Daan, Ph.D. The therapy is based on their discovery of the switchpoint (SP) and how circadian clocks are reset when a person is exposed to light before or after that point. Four National Institute of Mental Health doctors recently developed a highly specific, structured light therapy schedule, based on the earlier research. The Lewy-Daan approach is more generalized, but both approaches yield good results, according to studies.

Like food therapy, pretrip light strategies require self-discipline. You will require light exposure when those around you on home time (HT) are asleep, and you will need darkness when normally you would be exposed to sunlight at midday. To be successful, once you begin light therapy, you must follow *every step* and do it at the correct time. If your pretrip schedule absolutely precludes your following our recommendations, you should consider waiting until your travel day to begin—and accept the fact that your jet lag will last longer as a result.

Prepare by planning how and where you will be exposed to light when it's still dark outdoors and, conversely, how and where you will maintain total darkness when it is noon in HT.

Some sources of artificial light: While natural sunlight is always the best and brightest light source, effective artificial substitutes include the following:

- *Bright indoor light in your home or office,* at shopping malls, or in public buildings is a possibility. Your choices should reflect the likelihood of middle-of-the-night HT applications of light.

- *Standard incandescent or fluorescent lamps* facing a white reflective surface, such as a piece of paper or a white wall, provide adequate indirect bright light.

- *Portable light boxes or light visors,* designed specifically for changing circadian rhythms, are another reliable source of artificial light, although transporting them may be awkward.

Ways to achieve darkness: Experts recommend using an opaque, black-cloth eye mask that lets in no light for darkest periods. If such periods occur at a time when you would normally be in bed, you'll have no problem. If, however, they occur when you are normally awake and functioning in HT, plan to be in a place where you can be in total dark, preferably using an eyeshade, for at least the most critical three to four hours.

To move around in the darkest period, switch from eyeshade to dark glasses *without* turning on a light. Don't take unnecessary risks, however: if you have difficulty seeing with the very dark glasses, you should err on the side of safety, knowing the outcome of your program will be affected.

A word of caution: Don't use sunglasses during the most intense light exposure time, but do look at any light source indirectly. Bright, indirect light—whether sunlight or artificial—suffices.

Earlier we mentioned the 4 A.M. human switchpoint (SP), the dividing time between delaying and advancing your biological clocks. The SP can be used as a clock-setting mechanism: Should you, for some reason, be exposed to bright light before three or four hours of your SP, your clock will be delayed. Conversely, bright light exposure anytime for 3–4 hours after your switchpoint advances your clock. The closer that light exposure is to the SP, the more intense the effect: should you experience bright light during the night at the wrong time, it will set your progress back. The SP gives a good clue to travelers: flying east, you want bright light after 4 A.M. for several hours (early morning, just when you wake up at 6 A.M.). Flying west, you want bright light before the switchpoint, or as late in the day as possible without interrupting your sleep schedule.

Remember: Flying **East** = **advance** clock = **earlier** waking and bedtimes = light exposure **after** switchpoint. Flying **West** = **delay** clock = **later** waking and bedtimes = light exposure **before** switchpoint.

Pretrip Food Strategies

On the Fourth Day Before Your Trip
According to the Ehret diet, this is a feast day (high-protein, high-calorie breakfast and lunch; high-carbohydrate dinner and snacks). Abstain from xanthines (caffeinated coffee or tea or any caffeine-containing product) *except* between 3 P.M. and 5 P.M. home time (HT).

On the Third Day Before Your Trip
Ehret's diet: Fast day (low-calorie, low-carbohydrate menu—eight hundred calorie limit—from clear soups, juices, salads, and other "neutral" foods). Abstain from xanthines (caffeinated coffee or tea or any caffeine-containing product) *except* between 3 P.M. and 5 P.M. home time (HT).

Wurtman's recommendations: Initially, your body will continue to prepare for meals on the HT schedule when you are trying to eat on destination time (DT). Pay extra attention to eating energy- versus sleep-inducing foods at such times. For instance, if you are eating a breakfast on DT when on HT it would be dinnertime, eat a high-protein and low-carbohydrate meal to offset the naturally drowsy feelings and time cues you get when your stomach is readying for dinner.

Wurtman reminds us, too, that the mind is keenest during the first few hours of wakefulness and thus is most impervious to the effects of food. Later in the day, when the body clocks are winding down, the mind and body are most vulnerable to the effects of food. Pay extra attention, therefore, to lunches, dinners, and snacks.

General recommendations: What to eat for *eastbound travelers:* high-energy foods at breakfast and lunch and calming, sleep-inducing foods at dinner to advance clock. What to eat for *westbound travelers:* carbohydrate breakfast (to encourage you to sleep later), followed by high-energy lunch, afternoon snack, and dinner to delay clock. (See appendix A for meal and snack ideas.)

Eastbound timing: Eat one hour earlier each day until you advance enough to reach normal DT mealtimes. For example, flying east across seven time zones—if you normally eat breakfast at 7 A.M. HT (2 P.M. DT), eat an hour earlier each successive day until you "catch up" to breakfast at 7 A.M. DT. Do this for all meals.

Westbound timing: Subtract, or delay, one hour each day until you reach normal DT mealtimes.

Pretrip Activity Strategies

On the Third Day Before Your Trip
Along with light and dark, activity and rest—determinants of your sleep-wake cycle—are the most important external zeitgebers, which we talked about in chapter 1, in resetting your body's clocks. When to be active and when to rest are easily determined: whenever your anti–jet lag strategy calls for light exposure, you must be active, especially during the most intense light exposure period. Rest or sleep during your light avoidance, or dark, period. In adapting your sleep-wake cycle, you must be active at times when others may be sleeping, or vice versa. Fulfilling this out-of-sync pretrip schedule is feasible only with self-discipline and support from family, friends, and co-workers.

To live on a schedule very different from those operating on home time (HT), we suggest that you reduce all unnecessary noise where you sleep; turn off the telephone; make the bedroom as dark as possible, using opaque window shades (or dark eyeshades) or drapes; and advise family and friends not to disturb your rest-sleep periods. Similarly, for activity periods (when those around you may be sleeping), devise in advance active strategies such as exercises you can do quietly and activities that engage you mentally, including work that interests you or fast-paced reading. If you will be traveling with another person, devise a cooperative strategy so that you can reinforce each other as you adapt. Remember: If you find it impossible to sleep at all or for only part of your sleep-rest phase, remaining inactive in dark surroundings is as effective, although not as much so, as eight hours of sleep.

Force yourself to be active when your schedule calls for activity. For instance:

- During the remainder of the active period, move whenever you feel as though you're tiring, and keep your mind engaged by doing or reading something lively or that requires your concentration. There is some evidence, according to recent studies, that spontaneous activity is even more effective than planned activity. If you're in an active phase, take advantage of opportunities for spontaneous activities that may arise.
- Do not be active—mentally or physically—when you should be resting, or sedentary and mentally disengaged if you need to be active. Rest or activity at the wrong times

will have the opposite effect of what you
desire.

Pretrip Food Strategies

On the Second Day Before Your Trip
According to the Ehret diet, this is a feast
day (high-protein breakfast and lunch and
high-carbohydrate dinner). Abstain from
xanthines except between 6 P.M. and 11 P.M.,
then consume only sparingly.

Continue to move mealtimes an hour later
or earlier than the day before, depending on
which direction you are flying.

Pretrip Activity Strategies

On the Second Day Before Your Trip
Repeat the same schedule as on the third day
before your trip (see page 55), advancing
your waking and bedtimes two hours (eastbound) or delaying your waking and bedtimes two hours (westbound).

Pretrip Food Strategies

On the Day Before Your Trip
According to the Ehret diet, this is a fast day
(low-calorie, low-carbohydrate, low-fat meals

and a maximum of eight hundred calories for the day). Coffee, tea, cola, and other xanthines are permitted only between 6 P.M. and 11 P.M. eastbound. And they are permitted only in the morning westbound.

Continue to move mealtimes an hour later or earlier than the day before, depending on which direction you are flying.

Pretrip Activity Strategies

On the Day Before Your Trip
Continue advancing your waking and bedtimes an hour earlier than the day before (eastbound) or delaying your waking and bedtimes until you are waking and sleeping on destination time (westbound).

Packing and Logistics

18. Assemble a contingency kit to carry on board.
A kit stocked with toiletries and other items to meet various contingencies of air travel can help you combat jet lag and other discomforts of a long flight. Our list covers only items having to do with jet lag and general health and comfort while in flight. You will undoubtedly want to add to it your

own list of items (such as a one-day change of clothes, in case your luggage is lost). Here's our checklist, by category:

Eyes

- **eye drops:** If your eye doctor hasn't recommended a particular brand, there are nonprescription solutions to soothe dry, tired eyes.
- **wetting solution** and **contact lens case:** Wearers of contact lenses may fare better wearing **eyeglasses** when in-flight because of the dry cabin air.
- **wraparound dark glasses:** These can be regular or disposable variety, to be worn along with your normal dark glasses to intensify darkness.
- **eye mask:** Total blackout masks, available from drugstores and catalogs.
- **sunglasses that offer broad-spectrum UVA/UVB protection:** Glasses should be dark green or gray for the most effective ultraviolet screening, say Graber and Siegel in *Traveler's Medical Companion*, and should state percentage of UVA *and* UVB rays filtered. They recommend brands that adhere to American National Standards Institute's requirement that glasses labeled as UV filters must screen out 99 percent of UVB rays.
- **light visor:** This optional item, used by some frequent flyers to battle jet lag, is a battery-operated hat outfitted with a visor that emits bright light downward, onto the wearer but not

directly into the eyes. Relatively expensive (any-where from $150 to $350, with some rentals available at lower prices), this can be awkward to carry when traveling, but it is said to have a high success rate for those using light therapy.

Ears

- **earplugs:** These should be effective enough to quash surface noises, but not emergency an-nouncements over the public-address system.
- **sugarless chewing gum:** This will help relieve ear blockage, but use *only on takeoff and land-ing*. Chewing gum during your flight allows you to swallow too much air, which adds to the stom-ach discomfort created by gases expanding in your stomach from low air pressure (see page 31 for more on cabin air pressure).

Medicinal

- **analgesics** (whatever general-purpose pain re-liever you take for headaches)
- **antihistamine, decongestant, or commer-cially prepared combination:** These are available in over-the-counter or prescription forms to manage the congested nasal passages and/or sneezing associated with allergies, colds, and such. Also, many travelers use drowsiness-causing antihistamines as sleep aids when fly-ing. Check with your medical practitioner before you do this.

- **motion sickness medication:** Dramamine and Bonine are two leading brand-name pills, and scopolamine is available in patch form. Ginger, an herb that has long been used to calm an upset stomach, is available in capsule or candy form in health food stores.

- **bismuth salicylate:** This settles upset stomach and can help alleviate diarrhea. Pepto-Bismol is one brand name; it comes in liquid or tablet form. Pepcid and Zantac are also available without a prescription for short-term use.

- short-acting **sleeping pills** (if you and your doctor have agreed to follow this course of jet lag combat). (See box on page 64.)

- **candy (sugarless), cough drops, or lozenges:** These can help relieve and moisturize a sore throat and/or cough from allergies, a cold, or dry cabin air. Since sugar is a simple carbohydrate that can derail your food strategy if taken at the wrong time, sugarless varieties are recommended.

Orthopedic

- **lumbar pillow:** This thin, contoured back pillow helps ensure good posture throughout the flight and is a travel necessity for anyone with back problems, since most airline seats are not contoured properly and hold your back in a difficult and unhealthy position. (Think of the stiffness and pain—two of jet lag's troublesome side effects—you can help prevent.) Drug and surgical supply stores carry these, as do many chiropractors.

- **neck pillow:** This inflatable collar-shaped pillow supports your head while you doze (or try to) in a sitting position. *Remember:* Minimizing the disruption to your sleep-wake cycle is one of the best ways to prevent jet lag.

Skin Care

- **moisturizer** to rehydrate dry skin caused by cabin air.
- **sunscreen,** with an SPF of at least 15, since it is possible to absorb harmful ultraviolet rays through airplane windows.
- **lip balm,** preferably with an SPF factor, to prevent lips from chapping or getting sunburned.
- **saline spray**: This nonmedicated nasal moisturizer, available in squeeze bottles from drugstores, helps flush allergens from your nose while keeping it moist, so that you avoid the irritation and burning that result from too dry air. Moist nasal passages also help deflect cold and other germs.

Personal Hygiene

- **toothbrush, toothpaste, and breath spray:** These are obviously handy for refreshing yourself in flight.
- **razor, shaving cream**
- **hairbrush or comb**

- **washcloth or antibacterial wet wipes:** These help cleanse hands and face of germs.
- **facial tissues**

Miscellaneous

- **travel alarm or watch with an alarm:** Either is important for self-administered anti–jet lag light and food therapies.
- **personal tape player and several favorite tapes** for relaxation or mental engagement.
- **slippers:** These—especially soft, foldable ones or slipper socks that can be rolled in your luggage—are great substitutes for your shoes on a long flight, especially when you are trying to sleep. You will eliminate the discomfort of tight-fitting shoes when your legs and feet swell from prolonged sitting in a thin air environment.
- **self-adhesive badge or nametag:** You can stick the tag on your collar or sweater with printing big enough for an attendant to read at a five-foot distance. Print a polite message, such as "Please do not disturb. Wake only for landing."

19. Carry snacks on board.

The anti–jet lag diet therapy boxes explain the ins and outs of what foods to eat at what times on your trip, for optimum sleepiness or alertness, depending on when and in what direction you plan to fly. In many cases, eating airline food selectively at times pertinent to your (rather than the airline's) schedule will get you by. There are exceptions, however. So if your anti–jet lag approach suggests you'll need food at a time when the airline may not be serving, plan to take along your own snacks—some high in protein, others high in carbohydrates. As Judith Wurtman, Ph.D., explains in *Managing Your Mind and Mood Through Food,* it takes relatively small amounts of food—under two ounces usually—to fire up or crank down the appropriate brain chemicals in order to initiate sleep or alertness, so snacks do not have to be loaded with calories. Stay away from fatty foods because they are difficult to digest and will keep you awake if you are trying to sleep.

Suggestions for high-protein, alertness-producing foods and high-carbohydrate, sleep-inducing foods appear in appendix A.

The Pros and Cons of Jet Lag Drug Therapy

Whether they are by prescription or over-the-counter (OTC), drugs used to treat jet lag's effects aim at one goal: promoting sleep. But, there is no evidence that either OTC drugs or prescription-only sleeping pills help directly to reset the body's clocks.

Drug therapy to counteract jet lag is controversial.

Since almost all antihistamines produce

drowsiness as a side effect, they are the principal OTC drugs used by travelers for offsetting jet lag. Antihistamines can cause a
range of other side effects, including a hangover and "fuzzy" thinking once they wear
off—at a time when most travelers need to
be alert. Some physicians feel that antihistamines carry too many side effects to be
used for other than their intended purpose of
lessening allergic reactions. Others feel that
using an antihistamine for a day or two during long-distance travel is less harmful than
sustained loss of sleep.

Some travelers prefer taking prescription-
only, short-acting hypnotics—sleeping pills
or sedatives—to lessen jet lag. These drugs,
which take several hours rather than days or
weeks to clear from the body, are generally
hangover-free. Hypnotics work by suppress-
ing central nervous system (CNS) function,
which puts them off limits to those suffering
from pulmonary, liver, and heart ailments,
and those who are pregnant or taking
various medications, including antianxiety
drugs or other sedatives. The combination of
a hypnotic with alcohol, another CNS de-
pressant, can be fatal.

Three short-acting hypnotics lead the list
of drugs prescribed for limited, one- or
two-day use by travelers. Two—triazolam
(Halcion) and lorazepam (Ativan)—are benzodiazepines, the most popular class of sleeping pill in the United States since the 1960s.
Each is absorbed by the body quickly, a plus

for the passenger who wants to fall asleep on schedule while airborne or during the first one or two nights at a destination. Of the two, triazolam has a shorter half-life (the time it takes the drug to be excreted by the body) of three to five hours, while lorezapam can take from eight to twenty-five hours to be excreted. Benzodiazepines suppress the deepest stages of sleep while improving your lighter sleep stage. They tend to promote uninterrupted sleep and limit your ability to remember any awakenings you might experience. *While benzodiazepines have fewer side effects than their predecessors, they are nonetheless addictive when abused, can cause anxiety and rebound insomnia at withdrawal, and are intended to be used and are efficacious only for up to ten days, preferably for one or two days at a time.* A dosage of 15 mg or less is the maximum strength needed by travelers (and the elderly are cautioned to use less, since hypnotics affect them harder).

The newest short-acting sedative, touted as the hypnotic having the fewest side effects yet, is zolpidem (Ambien), which is literally in a class by itself. When it received FDA approval in 1993, this imidazopyridine compound marked the first chemically new class of sleeping pills in thirty years. Clinical tests and early use support its claims of leaving little or no daytime drowsiness, memory loss, rebound insomnia, or tolerance, and only limited potential for physical dependency. The drug hasn't been in use long enough for researchers to determine whether there may be long-term side effects. Zolpidem permits deeper sleep than benzodiazepines.

The downside to using most short-acting hypnotics is the potential for temporary memory loss, a serious side effect. This anterograde amnesia—known also as *travelers' amnesia*—is common enough to make the use of these drugs as a jet travel antidote controversial. Documented cases show that passengers who have consumed alcohol, even in small amounts, in combination with a short-acting hypnotic have experienced a walking blackout in which they may land, deplane, collect luggage, and even rent a car and drive to a hotel without being able to recall a single incident of their postdrug activity. Doctors believe that anterograde amnesia, which generally lasts for the duration of the drug's half-life, may be a result of dosage and use patterns, since it is not a side effect experienced by all users.

If you elect to use drug therapy as an adjunct to natural efforts to combat jet lag, these commonsense guidelines should prevail: Discuss drug therapy (and any other medications you may be taking) in advance with your doctor. Take short-acting hypnotics in as low a dosage as possible to still be effective. Take them for a maximum of several days. Use them only on longer flights (four-plus hours), where jet lag may be more pronounced. Never mix them with alcohol or

another sedative. Be sure to get your own
prescription; don't ever borrow a friend's.

---

20. Bring your own bottled water.

To avoid the dehydration created by the dryness
of pressurized cabin air—and the resultant muscle fatigue and general sleepiness—you should
drink no less than eight ounces of water or juice
(not coffee, tea, alcohol, or carbonated sodas) every
hour of your flight. If the airplane is full—as many
transoceanic or other long-distance flights often
are—you probably will not be able to keep up with
this requirement simply because of the sheer
number of people the attendants must serve. Frequently, too, the beverage service on such flights
runs out of bottled water during the course of the
flight.

You need not haul eight bottles on board, but
bring enough to augment what you're likely to get
at meal or beverage service times. A number of
bottled water companies package in soft plastic
eight-ounce bottles. Or bring several twenty-
ounce plastic bottles with resealable sports caps.

21. Start adjusting to your destination one to five days before you fly.

Whether you plan to beat jet lag using diet therapy, light therapy, activity therapy, or a combi-

nation of all three (which we recommend), start living as much of your eating and activity schedules as is possible as though you were already at your destination. (There's no hard and fast rule on how far in advance of your trip to start changing your schedule; in this book, however, we begin three to five days before a trip. Obviously the fewer time zones traveled, the less the need for a long lead time.) As always, the westbound traveler can get by with a bit less lead time than the eastbound one, who is flying toward the shorter day. But anything helps—even a day's adjustment is better than none at all.

22. Set your watch for the new time zone.
We've mentioned the importance of internal and external time cues in resetting your body's circadian clock. Becoming mentally adjusted to a later or earlier time is a large part of the jet lag battle. By setting a second watch to the new time a day or two before you leave, you will be giving your body another important time cue that supports the change.

How Some Frequent Flyers Minimize Travel Discomforts

Frequent flyers often have neither the home time to pretreat jet lag nor enough destination time to get over it before they travel elsewhere or back to their starting point. In fact, experts agree that when trips are so compact—such as a four-day round trip to Europe or the Pacific Rim countries from the United States—it may be best to skip jet lag adaptation altogether.

Some executives and diplomatic travelers wear two watches, says author Don Kowet in *The Jet Lag Book*. One watch is set to home time, on which the traveler continues to eat, sleep, and be active. The other is set to local, or destination, time for ease in scheduling or making appointments. With this strategy, business is conducted during "overlap time"— a time when the traveler normally would be alert and conducting business at home that coincides with business time at the destination.

Alternatively, they do what John H. Greist, M.D., and Georgia L. Greist, authors of *Fearless Flying,* call "the fast-in, fast-out" trip.[4] Using this approach, the traveler flies to the destination, works quickly to finish the project or meeting, then jets home again before jet lag hits. Under some such schedules, however, experts say you should still expect your body to experience a one- to two-day upset, just from the rigors of travel.

Business travelers can beat the bad news of jet travel by combining a variety of strategic travel tips, suggests National Institute of Mental Health's Dan A. Oren, M.D., a leading jet lag researcher and a coauthor of

[4]Chicago: Nelson-Hall Publishers, 1981.

Beating Jet Lag.[5] His recommendations include a) checking with your doctor to see if a sleep medication would be helpful for the few critical nights; b) arranging meetings at times when you would normally be awake and alert at home; c) scheduling a block of time following your return to catch up on missed sleep.

Frequent flyer business travelers interviewed by *Nation's Business* (July 1994) suggest the following:

- *staying away from highly processed foods, sweets, and alcohol* to avoid sugar highs and lows (and keeping in mind the tenets of the diets we mention here when eating meals and snacks).

- *avoiding work while airborne* in favor of more restful, personally entertaining activity such as recreational reading, electronic games, or music.

- *choosing a flight to maximize airborne rest or sleep*, with a landing time that ensures a better night's sleep at the destination, before the business meeting. Where no such convenient flights are available, scheduling a brief—one- to two-day—stopover en route to "decompress" is suggested.

- *choosing a seat wisely in advance* of the

[5]New York: Henry Holt, 1993.

flight to ensure maximum body space and
leg room.

- *dressing casually* in clothes that are comfortable for flying rather than appropriate
for the business presentation ahead.

Finally, frequent business flyers need to
take a psychological approach to beating jet
lag on quick and frequent trips. In *Traveler's
Medical Companion*, authors Graber and
Siegel suggest that you

- *follow a stress management program,* and
combine it with isometrics once airborne
(the latter improves circulation while relieving the physical stress and mental tension of high-pressure travel).
- *walk frequently* (in the plane and on the
ground).
- *pack half* of the clothes and supplies you
think you'll need.
- *pack extras of any important business doc-
uments in your carry-on,* to offset the
trauma of lost luggage.
- *anticipate time shifts* by adjusting at home
as much as possible. (If that's impossible,
they advise you to eat lightly, avoid alcohol, and use caffeine to advantage.)
- *avoid all alcohol if you are taking a short-
acting sleeping pill* (see pages 65–67).
- *carry with you some tedious projects* from
your in-box that can be done during a flight
delay.

- *take recreational "junk" reading for before bed or to peruse on the plane.*
- *build and maintain a file of friends, restaurants, and local activities you enjoy when you travel to a particular destination.*
- *keep flexible and maintain a sense of humor.*

Takeoff: Travel Day

For light therapy, follow the time on your travel watch. If you have not yet caught up or backed up to your DT, continue to re-set by an hour each day. Go to sleep and rise at your regular times—for example 11 P.M. and 6 A.M.—travel-watch time. Where necessary wear dark glasses or an eyemask, especially between the hours of 10 P.M. and 1 or 2 A.M. (when you need to be in the darkest period). Use light—even the overhead reading light in the plane—if travel time is between 6 A.M. and 6 P.M. Similarly, you'll need to be extra vigilant and keep a mask on until it's 6 A.M. travel-watch time, even if others are moving about.

If you have not had an opportunity to start your anti–jet lag adaptation earlier, start by setting your watch to DT and living by your destination's light schedule. You'll be following the same schedule of light and light avoidance as those around you who adapted earlier, but your jet lag will hit you harder, taking you a longer time to adjust fully.

Pretrip Food Strategies

On Your Travel Day

According to the Ehret diet, on this day you break your fast with a high-protein, high-calorie breakfast. Hereafter, switch your meals to normal times, foods, and serving sizes.

Wurtman's recommendations are as follows:

Eastbound: Eat your normal breakfast. At lunch, eat a larger, dinnerlike (carbohydrate-intensive) meal both in portion and type of food. Drink your last cup of coffee or tea for the next few hours. For your midday snack, have carbohydrates if you are on a night flight and will be sleeping most of the time. If you are flying in early evening, your rhythms will have peaked by 4 P.M. or 5 P.M., says Wurtman, so consume coffee or tea and appropriate high-protein foods to help you stay awake. If you will be boarding in early evening, eat a high-carbohydrate dinner *before* you board to prime you for sleep once you take off.

Westbound: Sleep as late as you can. Eat a small breakfast, high in protein to delay your clock. End coffee consumption until late afternoon.

Move mealtimes an hour earlier (east-bound) or later (westbound) than the day be-fore. If your travel day mealtimes have not yet coincided with the eating times you'll be following at your destination.

Pretrip Light Strategies

On Your Travel Day

Repeat the same schedule as on the day before your trip (see page 58).

Since your travel will dictate your sched-ule today, you will need to be especially vig-ilant about light exposure and light avoidance for the right length of time and at the correct time of day.

Pretrip Activity Strategies

On Your Travel Day

If your waking and bedtimes (eastbound) have not yet "caught up" to those at your des-tination, advance each one hour. Delay wak-ing and bedtimes (westbound) one hour each, unless you are already "backed up" to desti-nation time.

If your travel will begin during your rest-sleep phase, try to minimize activity and re-sume rest as soon as you board the plane. If you are in your active phase, move around as long as you can before boarding. Once seated for takeoff, be certain your mind is engaged (reading, writing, or talking with rowmate) and active.

23. Dress comfortably.

When planning your in-flight wardrobe, remember the confined space of a plane. Remember, too, that those days are gone when air passengers dressed to the nines. Today, dressing for comfort should be your main consideration. Your wardrobe should ideally consist of loose-fitting, comfortable clothing, with cottons preferred over synthetic fabrics that don't breathe as well. The loose fit will accommodate any swelling or bloating caused by thin air, low cabin pressure, and long periods of sitting. Such clothing will also encourage better rest or sleeping.

Wear comfortable shoes. Women should consider leaving high heels at home (or at least in the suitcase), favoring low, cushioned shoes instead. No shoes should be tight: remember that feet are apt to swell in flight. Wear cotton socks rather than synthetic varieties; panty hose are not a good idea for women since the elasticity can grow tight during flight, due to swelling caused from lower air pressure. You can kick off your shoes once you're airborne, substituting cotton socks for the slippers we recommended (thus saving space in your carry-on).

CHAPTER 3

Beating Jet Lag
While In-Flight

Because you started altering your eating and light exposure cycles even before boarding the plane, your body clock is already on the way to resetting itself. Once airborne, the three therapies of food, light, and action move to center stage, where they should remain until after your arrival and after your jet lag disappears. Defeating jet lag will depend on how closely you follow the instructions and timing recommended in these three critical areas.

All other tips are secondary to food, light, and action, although none is unimportant. In fact, any measure you take aloft to overcome discomforts or assaults on your body's systems will better prepare you to combat jet lag at your destination.

In-Flight Light Strategies

Continue to have light exposure in the morning (travel-watch time) flying east, and shade and dark in late afternoon and evening (after 6 P.M. travel-watch time). Those flying west need to have shade or dark in mornings, with as much light as possible in late afternoon, up until 6 P.M.

Remember to have eyeshades as well as dark glasses readily available at your seat. If it's daylight outside during your light-avoidance stage, pull down the window shade and turn off the reading light. Keep the dark glasses where you can find them easily. If you must walk to the lavatory, switch to dark glasses, keeping eyes closed while making the switch. In the light phase, do the opposite: put up the shade and keep on the reading light (or have a light visor in place and operational).

If you have scheduled a stopover, keep on the same light-dark schedule.

On a short stopover where you must leave the plane briefly, seek well-lighted areas near airport displays, in hallways, and by ticket counters. Seek darkest areas in less well-lit corners of unused airport lounges near your deplaning site. (If you are resting, be sure to set your watch alarm to avoid sleeping through the boarding call.)

On a longer stopover, including an overnight stay, proceed on your schedule, wearing sunglasses and/or eyeshades for the necessary time. Wearing dark glasses will not preclude your moving around, but the light-avoidance period—if you want to avoid setbacks—typically should be a quiet time, free of activity.

In-Flight Food Strategies

Ehret's diet: After your high-protein breakfast and before landing, eat foods that will help you fulfill your light and activity therapies. (Remember the formula: proteins for alertness, carbohydrates for drowsiness and sleep.)

Wurtman's recommendations: If your strategy calls for sleeping on the plane, it's okay to drink one to two glasses of wine to make you sleepy. (If you do, compensate for the diuretic effect by drinking more water and using your saline nasal spray to help offset dehydration's effects.) She suggests asking to be awakened for breakfast, which on Europe-bound flights is usually served ninety minutes before landing. If you eat, go easy on carbohydrates (which can be real knockouts if you have not slept well on the flight). If you are traveling farther east than

Europe, skip breakfast aloft and maintain your sleep schedule.

General recommendations: Follow an in-flight meal and snack plan that consists of proteins when you need to be alert and carbohydrates when you need to wind down and sleep. Avoid all fats and, unless specifically called for, alcohol and caffeine.

If you have ordered in advance high-protein or high-carbohydrate meals to meet your requirements, have backups to the airline meals. Since you may be sleeping when meals are served, you run the risk of missing your special meals altogether (and special orders often do not materialize on the plane).

Eat small portions. It's harder to digest food while you are sitting. And, as Wurtman points out, it doesn't take more than an ounce or two of protein or carbohydrates to set into action the food/brain effect you are seeking.

If you are eating a high-protein meal that contains a mix of carbohydrates and proteins, be certain to eat protein first (for example, a slice of meat or a wedge of low-fat cheese before a roll) if you are intending to stay alert. Wurtman's work shows that even a small amount of protein eaten first initiates brain production of the alertness neurotransmitters that also help block the brain's manufacture of sleep-inducing serotonin. (The reverse is true—carbohydrates before proteins—if you are planning to sleep.)

If you have scheduled a stopover, use the time on the ground to advantage if it coincides with a mealtime at your destination.

If you are having difficulty staying awake when you need to, Wurtman suggests a small snack of a protein or a "neutral food" like fruit. The goal is to keep your metabolic rate up because then your digestion will need to work, which will make sleeping difficult.

In-Flight Activity Strategies

Continue your sleep-wake schedule to coincide with your light therapy. Stay active until you enter the light-avoidance stage. Do in-seat exercises or crossword puzzles, read stimulating material, or talk with your rowmate. When it's safe to do so, stroll the aisle periodically, doing stretching exercises along the way.

If you have scheduled a stopover, keep on your sleep-wake schedule as much as you can.

On a short stopover where you must leave the plane briefly, use the time to walk briskly through well-lighted airport corridors, if in your active phase, or find a dimly lighted airline boarding area where you can sit to rest. (Be sure not to sleep through reboarding. A watch alarm will help.)

On a longer stopover, including an overnight stay, proceed on your sleep-wake schedule.

24. Put pillows in their place.

Unless you've brought your own neck pillow, you may want to pick up an airline pillow (and blanket) as you board. If you've brought the contoured lumbar pillow, as we suggested, put that in place before you buckle into your seat. (In lieu of that, bring along a small towel rolled up and bound with rubber bands, and place in the seat back at the base of your spine.)

25. Establish your turf and conditions.

To maximize leg room under the seat in front of you, place as much of your carry-on luggage as possible in the overhead bins. Keep at hand any part of your carry-on kit that you'll need soon: eyeshades, a particular snack, or that Velcro-backed badge noting "Please do not disturb. Wake only for landing." Position your badge where the attendant is most likely to see it. Then, even if you don't get to speak with your attendant before you sleep, you'll be wearing your wishes prominently. (Some airlines offering transcontinental flights have been experimenting with "sleeper service" in their business or first-class sections. The flyer eats a light meal served in the airport's airline club, then boards to a reclining seat equipped with a pillow and comforter. In-flight sleep amenities include no lights, no noise, and no meal carts. If you're on a hectic business schedule, you may want to look into this service.)

26. Set your watch for the new time zone, if you didn't do it earlier.

Tuning all parts of your life—mental and physical—to your destination time is essential to getting the jump on jet lag. If you were unable to begin your anti–jet lag strategy in the days before you left, now is the time to do it. Remember: If you are taking time-sensitive medication such as insulin, beta-blockers, or birth control pills, keep a second watch set to home time, the schedule you should continue to follow for your medication.

27. Push those relaxation buttons.

While you await takeoff, put on your headphones and listen to the relaxing tapes you brought along.

It's also a good time for doing the deep-breathing exercises we mentioned in chapter 2, especially if you are an anxious flyer. If your sleep-wake schedule calls for resting immediately after takeoff, these relaxation efforts will put you in a frame of mind conducive to sleep and they will also signal your rowmate(s) that you will be resting rather than talking on your flight. (Of course, you might also want to mention to the person next to you that you're following a sleep schedule, so you will not be talking or eating during much of the flight.)

28. Clear your ears.
If your ears are apt to clog on the plane's ascent or descent (likely if you are currently suffering from allergies or a chronic sinus condition), just prior to takeoff is a good time to use your nasal decongestant spray. (If you use a decongestant pill, you should have taken it already so that it's effective by the time you take off.)

True, decongestants are not strictly "natural" preventive strategies, but they have their place in your in-flight regimen, as well as yawning, swallowing frequently, and chewing gum (the latter, as we already mentioned, only during ascent and descent). These actions temporarily contract your throat muscles, which opens your eustachian tubes (the canals from ear to throat that are blocked by inflammation when you have allergies, sinus troubles, or a cold). Don't wait until your ears clog to take corrective action: the more the blockage takes hold, the harder it will be to clear.

If you do not have a sinus condition or cold, here are two corrective maneuvers you can try.

Valsalva's maneuver: This involves closing your mouth, pinching your nostrils shut, and blowing your cheeks out as if you are blowing up a balloon. This can result in light-headedness (as such, *it is not a good procedure for those with heart conditions or blood vessel problems*).

Frenzel's maneuver: This is the alternative that anyone can try. According to the authors of *Fearless Flying*, here's what to do: Close your mouth and temporarily hold your breath. Pinch your nostrils shut, then contract the muscles of the floor of your mouth (as you would when swallowing) and swallow.

Using either maneuver, you should feel your ears "pop" and your hearing will clear. If not, repeat the procedure several times until it works. Follow this same procedure later on, as you descend.

29. Anticipate body changes.

Kick off your shoes, don those slippers or socks that you packed, and loosen your waistband. Not only will these actions help you relax more, they'll be helping your body adjust to the changes it undergoes at thirty thousand to forty thousand feet. Here are some of the effects of the high altitude on your body (suggestions to counter them appear in tips that follow):

- **dehydration:** The cabin air is pressurized to equalize air at 5,000 to 7,500 feet above sea level. This low pressure is dryer than air at sea level. Under these conditions, the mucous membranes around your eyes, nose, and mouth dry out, and with acceleration of the natural evaporation of body fluids caused by dry conditions, you can easily become dehydrated and, from there, fatigued.
- **strained breathing:** Low pressure carries less breathable oxygen, so your heart and lungs have to work harder to bring a sufficient supply into your blood and tissues.
- **disequilibrium:** The shift from high to lower air pressure while in-flight creates an imbalance between your insides and the outside environment, causing gases in your body—the average adult, according to Greist, holds between 150 and 500 cubic centimeters of gas in the digestive tract at any one time—to expand, thus creating the feeling of stomach and intestinal bloatedness.
- **edema:** Swelling in the extremities—legs, ankles, feet—happens when water and salt fluids from the blood leak from the capillaries into surrounding tissues. Edema of the feet and ankles is a common occurrence in those who sit for any length of time in a confined position, since gravity pulls fluids down.

- **compromised circulation:** Edema constricts blood circulation in the affected areas. Blood pressure by itself isn't adequate to return blood from the veins in the legs to the heart. It must be aided by a "milking action" of the calf and thigh muscles on deep veins in the leg, explains Greist, an impossibility in one who is immobile for any length of time, as in a long plane flight. The situation is made worse in a plane, where less oxygen is present and the body must work harder to move oxygen into the cells. Given these conditions, a person is prime for developing potentially dangerous blood clots. Once a clot forms, it can break loose (or embolize) in the veins of the legs—a condition called *phlebitis*— and flow upward through veins of the heart and into a lung, where it can become lodged in the pulmonary artery. This prevents your lung from working correctly, interferes with oxygen supply for the whole body, and can be fatal.

There are general health tips for offsetting those high altitude body changes that will also help you beat jet lag.

Stay Moist

30. Drink plenty of liquids.
Dehydration is an insidious process; it generally happens without our even being aware of it. You

know the dictum—drink at least eight ounces an hour of water or low-sugar fruit juices.

31. Shun alcohol and caffeine in-flight.

You already know that some of the anti–jet lag diets we've highlighted suggest points at which you'll benefit from a caffeinated beverage or food. Other than such an instance, it's best to entirely avoid caffeine products and alcoholic drinks.

Furthermore, you don't want to be battling an alcohol hangover while you're trying to minimize the effects of jet lag. It takes less time for alcohol to reach your bloodstream if you drink while flying. So two drinks in the air pressure of a typical jet cabin are equal to three at sea level. More attention also has been paid recently to added dangers of drinking red wines, sherry, or port in-flight, as these carry histamines, the allergens that can increase head congestion (and possibly ear problems when the plane descends and continued discomfort at your destination).

32. Use a saline nasal spray.

Keeping the mucous membranes of the nasal passages moist is one of your first (and best) lines of defense in fighting germs and allergens that may be circulating in the air of the plane. Unless you are on your sleep-rest schedule, use a saline nasal mist at least once an hour.

33. Suck on lozenges or hard candy.

Just as with the nasal passages, your throat needs to stay moist if you are to counteract the conditions that cause or worsen jet lag's effects. We recommend sugarless hard candy, not only because it is better for your teeth, but also because introducing sugar into your body at the wrong time can undermine the positive effects of the food therapy you are following. (On the other hand, if you're at the point of sleep-wake therapy that calls for alertness, a gumdrop or hard candy won't hurt. Avoid chocolate, though, which has too high a fat content to make digestion easy.)

34. Put your skin on a moisturizing and sun-protection schedule.

Maintaining healthy, moist skin gives your body a better line of defense against infection from cuts and scratches and protects it better against the ravages of the sun's harmful rays. Sustaining ultraviolet-B damage to your skin through the windows of an aircraft is not only possible, but at high altitudes where air is thinner it is more dangerous than the same exposure at sea level.

Start your flight with an application of moisturizer and sunblock with an SPF factor of at least 15. Many commercial products now combine moisturizing lotion with sunblock protection. Reapply the moisturizer after washing your hands during your flight and whenever your face feels dry.

35. Take frequent freshness breaks.

On one of your exercise walks to the lavatory, take your toiletry bag from the carry-on kit (the one where you've packed washcloth, face soap, toothbrush, toothpaste, and hairbrush). Splash your face with cold water (rinse off old moisturizer). Brush your teeth, reapply the moisturizer, and brush or comb your hair. If you skip a break to stay in your seat, using one of the moist towelettes you packed achieves some of the same freshening effects. This refreshing procedure is a helpful mental zeitgeber if you are switching from a sleeping to an activity cycle.

36. Keep your eyes and lips moist.

A long flight guarantees dry-eye problems, a situation usually exacerbated in those who wear contact lenses. Use the antidotes you've packed in your carry-on kit—hourly or more often if your eyes still feel irritated. Also, in the cabin's dry atmosphere, your eyes are apt to feel more comfortable if contact lenses are removed during the sleep-rest cycle. Hourly lip balm application is important, too. You can take care of sun protection at the same time if you've packed a lip balm that has an SPF factor.

Pamper Your Stomach

37. Give your digestive system a break.

Don't forget that while in-flight your digestive system is working under a great deal of stress from the disequilibrium of air pressure (and the dry air). You should already be following an anti–jet lag diet and should also be avoiding salty foods, starting with those traditional airline cocktail peanuts. Salt exacerbates the dry-air/dehydration problem. Go out of your way to avoid chocolate and any other foods high in fats (most kinds of chips and many nuts), since fats tax the digestive system, causing it to work overtime. Stay clear of highly acidic foods (tomatoes, oranges, grapefruit, and pineapple juice) and spicy foods.

Other digestive system punishments are any foods or drinks that produce gas, including carbonated drinks. Jean Carper, author of *Food: Your Miracle Medicine*, includes foods from the bean family and some other vegetables that contain oligosaccharide sugars (brussels sprouts, cauliflower, cabbage, dried beans and peas, onions, and soybeans); lactose, the sugar in milk and other dairy products (yogurt being the exception), especially gas producing for those with lactose intolerance; soluble fiber found in such foods as oat bran and apples; and, to less of a degree, most carbohydrates (rice being the exception).[1] Watch out,

[1]New York: HarperCollins, 1993.

too, for sorbitol, the low-calorie sweetener that, says Carper, is a "ferocious gas producer."

38. Deflate that gassy, bloated feeling.

You won't be able to totally eliminate gas and bloating in-flight, but you can moderate gaseousness by using a *carminative,* an agent that helps expel gas (mostly in burps, rather than flatulence). According to Carper, carminatives also have an antispasmodic and muscle-relaxing effect in the intestine. Foods with carminative properties include anise, basil, chamomile, dill, fennel seeds, garlic, peppermint, and sage. Ginger helps relieve gas as well as motion sickness. You may want to bring along a chamomile teabag (attendants will provide you with hot water), peppermint drops or candies, ginger cookies or ginger candies.

In deference to your rowmate, you may want to hold off on the garlic until you've landed. If all else fails, *Fearless Flying* authors call for any preparation containing simethicon (an ingredient in many antacid products), a silicon derivative that reduces the surface tension of gas bubbles in the stomach and allows them "to coalesce into larger bubbles more easily belched." This works for discomfort of only the stomach, not the large intestine. The best advice if all herbs and medications fail to relieve your gas is to move around.

Avoid Blood Clots, Edema, and Stiffness

39. Take an aspirin.
Studies show that aspirin en route, along with exercise, reduces the possibility of blood clots caused by long periods of immobility. Check with your doctor first, though, before you take an aspirin or two preceding a long flight.

40. Don't sit with your legs crossed.
Crossing your legs while sitting cuts off blood flow. In the limited space of most passenger seats in coach or economy class, crossing one's legs is not an option, but in the more spacious confines of first and business class, it pays to remember to keep your feet uncrossed and flat on the floor. (For spinal comfort, you may want to prop your feet on a book or knapsack to raise them slightly off the floor, still keeping your legs uncrossed.)

41. Exercise your calf muscles.
Here's an in-seat exercise that ought to keep your blood flowing upward and help you avoid what's become known as "economy-class syndrome." Start by contracting each of your calf muscles. Do this, recommend the Greists, by raising your toes

off the floor as far as is comfortable while keeping your heel down as a pivot point. Or lift your heel, while using the toe as a pivot. Do these exercises for twenty-five to thirty seconds per leg every five to ten minutes.

42. Take a walk.

Walking, stretching, and exercising, in general, are the best methods for avoiding blood clots on a flight. Try to walk the length of your seating section at least once an hour (excluding when you are in a sleep cycle, the airline beverage service is in progress, or the captain has the seat belt sign turned on). If you're a nervous flyer who prefers to stay in your seat, there are exercises for you, too. They range from isometrics to confined stretching (see next tip) and in-seat acupressure (see page 96).

43. After sleep, give your body a wake-up call.

In addition to swelling of legs, feet, ankles, and hands from inactivity while you're sleeping, other changes happen to your body. Notes jet lag specialist Ehret, your heartbeat drops ten to twenty beats per minute, lowering your temperature and allowing your muscles and joints to stiffen and lose elasticity and your conscious mind to become sluggish. To get yourself moving after a rest period, Ehret recommends these seven exercises, most of which can be done from your seat or in the aisle if you prefer not to move around the cabin. (Before starting any new exercise, clear them in advance with your medical practitioner.)

- *Take five deep breaths* to pump lungs full of oxygen and change air in bottom of lungs.
- *Stand on toes and stretch* for the ceiling five to ten times.
- *Slowly rotate shoulders in both directions:* left shoulder five times forward, five backward. Then rotate both simultaneously forward and backward. (This is also excellent for making a stiff back more limber and for offsetting pain in shoulder blade trigger points.)
- *Rotate head twice clockwise to the right,* twice counterclockwise to the left; repeat five times. Do not rotate in a full circle—it could cause damage to the neck nerves.
- *Bend backward from waist,* with chin pointed toward ceiling; repeat five times.
- *Rotate wrists and ankles,* twenty times each ten to right, ten to left.
- *Pull knees up* to waist, five times for each leg.

Personal Hygiene and Comfort

44. Wash your hands and don't touch your face.

The primary way that we contract colds and flu is by self-inoculation, the act of touching something or someone carrying the germ, then touching our eyes, nose, or mouth. On a long flight, where conditions are close and the dry air is working against your immune system's first lines of defense by drying out eyes and nasal passages, it's important to wash your hands often and to remind yourself to keep your hands away from your face.

45. Try acupressure to cure a variety of airplane-associated discomforts.

Acupressure, the healing art that uses finger pressure on acupuncture points and meridians of the body to release muscle pain and tension and improve circulation, has devoted followers in the frequent flyer ranks. As used in acupressure, a meridian is a human energy pathway that connects the various acupressure points and the internal organs. The points are actually pressure points, places on the body along a meridian with high levels of electrical conductivity. Among other things, self-administered airborne acupressure can be used to relieve motion sickness, anxiety, foot cramps, and neck or shoulder tension. Acupressurist Michael Reed Gach, author of *Acupressure's Potent Points,* explains how:[2]

- **motion sickness:** Press firmly with forefinger and middle finger on acupressure point P-6 (in the middle of the inner side of the forearm two and one-half finger widths above the wrist crease).
- **anxiety or fear:** Press on point GV-24.5 (directly between the eyebrows, in the indentation where the bridge of the nose meets the forehead) to calm the body and relieve nervousness. Or press on CV-17 (at the center of the breastbone, three thumb widths up from the base) to relieve nervousness, anxiety, and chest tension.
- **foot and ankle pain from swelling:** Press on K-3 (in the hollow midway between the protrusion of the inside anklebone and the Achilles' tendon, which joins the back of the calf to the back of the heel) or on the B-60 (opposite K-3 in the hollow between the outer anklebone and the Achilles' tendon).
- **neck and shoulder tension:** Using the first two fingers of either hand, press lightly on point TW-16 (indentation at base of skull, one to two inches in back of earlobe, depending on size of head).

Whenever acupressure techniques specify applying pressure, several minutes is the recommended duration.

[2]New York: Bantam Books, 1990.

46. Consider aromatherapy and herbal products.

A London aromatherapist, who employs the ancient art of scents to heal, recently undertook a study to test flight crews and other frequent travelers' reactions to aromatherapy products aimed at increasing flying comfort, and eliminating some of jet lag's effects. The scents used were to stimulate the participants while in-flight and to promote sleep once on the ground. A June 1995 *Town & Country* article reporting on the 1994 study's results indicated a 73 percent positive response from flight crews who felt the products were "extremely helpful." As a result, several British airlines are now giving aromatherapy kits to their first-class passengers.

Essential oils extracted from herbs have been used through the centuries to stimulate and sedate. One company manufactures a combination of herbal oils called "the Sleep Enhancer" (combining sandalwood and lavender) and "the Energizer" (mint and orange) in sprays for applying either to a flyer's pulse points or to the headrest of the airplane seat. There's no clinical proof that these remedies work, but given the strong link between mind and body, if either works for you, use it. Since herbals can cause allergic reactions, it's a good idea to try these at home, before you fly, to be certain you and they are compatible.

47. To induce sleep, try a homeopathic remedy.

A dilution of pulsatilla (windflower) is a homeopathic remedy for insomnia characterized by difficult sleep onset, according to Nancy Bruning and Corey Weinstein, M.D., writing in *Healing Homeopathic Remedies* (Dell Publishing, New York, 1996). Homeopathic medicine tries to stimulate the body's natural defenses through administration of a highly diluted substance that causes the same symptoms you are attempting to cure (their theory is "like cures like"). Therefore, a homeopathic treatment for sleeplessness is aimed at inducing sleeplessness. Homeopaths use the lowest effective doses, with every remedy highly diluted in water or alcohol. One homeopathic dose consists of a dilution (such as one part per million in a water or alcohol base) in drops (5–10), tablets (2–3), globules (2–3), or granules (15–20). For mild sleeplessness, Bruning and Weinstein recommend one dose of pulsatilla every six hours, repeated until symptoms disappear. Dilutions are mixed by homeopathic pharmacists to fixed recipes, and sold in homeopathic pharamacies, health food stores, and some supermarkets and pharmacies. Bruning and Weinstein also recommend trying passionflower, with or without the addition of valerian, to treat sleeplessness. Both herbals have been used through history as mild sedatives. The easiest form is a tea, using 1/2 to 1 tsp. of the dried herb(s) to a cup of boiling water, repeated every three to four hours as necessary.

Homeopathic treatments, like herbals, are drugs, and used in too concentrated a solution, many are toxic. For this reason, it is essential that you consult your doctor before adding homeopathic or herbal regimens to your anti–jet lag regimen.

Rest Wisely

48. Use presleep rituals from home.

When you're about to start your sleep or rest cycle, attune your mind to your schedule by repeating some of the same prebedtime habits—called *sleep hygiene*—that you follow at home. These can include drinking a bedtime glass of water; brushing your teeth; taking before-bed medications; washing your face; and applying moisturizer to your skin. Sleep hygiene also covers how we unwind our minds before sleep or rest. Do quiet activities in your seat that will disengage your mind. In other words, set aside that action-packed book you were reading and tune out the race-and-chase in-flight movie you might otherwise be tempted to watch. If you're listening to tapes, be sure the music is relaxing, not lively.

CHAPTER 4

What to Do Once You're There

The flight's over, you've deplaned, and if you started your anti–jet lag strategies before your trip, by now you should be operating just about normally. If you started adapting late—or not at all—you may feel as though you're about to die, or at least as if you want to lie down anywhere you can to sleep.

Even if you're feeling good, it's important to remember the statistics: untreated jet lag impairs judgment by as much as 20 percent the first day at a destination. Don't be surprised if your short-term memory fails, leaving you clueless when the car rental agency at your destination asks your home address. As we've noted before, jet lag disrupts both the mental and physical you. In *Overcoming Jet Lag*, author Charles Ehret notes that jet lag alters your reaction time, mental alertness, grip strength, and ability to calculate a math problem. Basic psychomotor performance—coordination and reflexes—can run out of sync from two days to two weeks, although most people are back to normal in five to ten days.

The worst feature of this body-clock adjustment period is its subtlety, which can be downright dangerous. "The trickiest period is right after arrival, when you think you're alert," writes Gerald A. Michaelson in the December 1994 *Success*. "That's when you lose things and accidents happen. Allow a day or two before driving a car, engaging in a serious business meeting, or making significant financial decisions."

Anticipate a more difficult adjustment if you have flown east. One study conducted in the early 1980s concluded that in the first thirty or forty hours after a westbound flight, biological rhythms shifted 20 to 80 percent more in phase—or coinciding more closely with destination time (DT)—than after an eastbound flight.[1]

Don't be alarmed if a traveling companion reacts to jet lag differently or bounces back from it sooner than you do. Jet lag expert Ehret compares different people to the different clocks in a store: they all tell time, but each is a little different. He predicts that most adults' heart rates will take five to six days (after adaptation begins) to adjust, uri-

[1]Donald Kowet, *The Jet Lag Book* (New York: Crown Publishers, 1983).

nary output up to ten days, and the gastrointestinal system, including bowels, up to twenty-four hours per zone crossed to readjust the body's elimination processes.

If your circadian clocks need additional resetting before you're fully operational on DT, our fundamental food, light, and action tips in special boxes throughout this chapter *must* be followed assiduously once you've arrived at your destination. This is when you are most apt to skimp or skip parts of these therapies.

Light Strategies at Your Destination

Travel Day: Upon Landing

- Maintain the light-dark schedule you have been following. On shorter trips east or west, crossing four or fewer time zones, you will be within a day or two of being fully adjusted to the light-dark schedule when you land, if you have followed the special tips in chapters 2 and 3. (Or you may already have acclimated to destination time [DT].)

- Even if you feel extraordinarily tired from the stresses of travel, fight the urge to nap in your daylight period. Go outside to seek light, if possible, and combine your outing with activity.

Food Strategies at Your Destination

Travel Day: Upon Landing

If you have started your resetting task prior to travel day, you should be close to eating on a destination time (DT) schedule. Therefore, follow your normal DT eating schedule (otherwise advance or delay meals until your schedule coincides with that of your destination).

- *Eat your meals when the natives do.*
- According to the Ehret diet, the first morning following your departure—bear in mind that, depending upon the flight schedule, you may still be airborne at this time—*eat a high-protein breakfast and lunch and a high-carbohydrate dinner.* This combination should help you fight fatigue and also help you stay awake until the normal bedtime on DT.
- According to the Wurtman diet, *eat all meals on DT.* (Be aware that you may be eating at times when your body is telling you that it's the middle of the night. And at odd times, such as in the very early morning or the middle of the night, you may become ravenous.

Eastbound: Breakfast and lunch are high-protein; dinners and snacks are high-carbohydrate. Proteins early in the day, according to DT, rev you up just as your home time (HT) habits are trying to slow you down. Carbohydrates late in the day DT slow you down just as HT habits are preparing you to be active. A drink with dinner is permitted (although wine can prolong jet lag). Eat a sweet snack one hour before bedtime DT. If you awaken in middle of the night, eat something sweet (low-fat candies, including jelly beans and gumdrops). Do not succumb to carbohydrate cravings before you're ready to go to sleep for the night. The cravings are your body's way of tricking you into sleep, explains Wurtman.

Westbound: Breakfast is high-carbohydrate. Follow with a high-protein lunch and dinner. It's okay to drink xanthine-containing beverages during the times of day you need to be awake.

Activity Strategies at Your Destination

Travel Day: Upon Landing

- Follow your normal schedule to coincide with normal mealtimes and sleep-wake times at your destination.
- *Stay active until your new bedtime.* Don't give in to the urge to sleep. If you find your energy flagging, walk briskly, jog, march in place, and get out in the daylight when you do.
- *Exercise fifteen to twenty minutes a day. Re-*

member: To help assure good sleep, exercise vigorously (until you raise your temperature two degrees) five to six hours before you want to sleep.

- *If it's time to be active, walk, take tours that engage your mind* (preferably outdoors, in daylight). Interact with other people. If you are in a resting phase before bedtime, do quiet activities, preferably indoors. Listen to the radio or taped music, watch a movie on television (but not an action-packed thriller), write a letter or a postcard, take a warm bath.

- *Be open to spontaneous activity,* which, studies show, can be even more effective than planned activity. Decide on the spur of the moment to walk to a local park, attend a fast-paced movie, or shop in a busy city center.

- *If you absolutely must nap,* be certain your traveling companion or the hotel operator awakens you in an hour or less; otherwise you will undo much of your anti–jet lag effort.

- *Go to bed when the natives do.* If you started your adjustment in the few days before you left home, you will find this an easier prospect. It will also be easier to sleep at normal DT if you have landed in the early to late evening rather than the morning.

- Research shows that *exaggerating such ex-*

ternal time cues as activity can help you adjust faster. Strive to keep a full activity schedule in these early hours after you land. Or if you are in a rest period, get to your destination lodging as soon and as quietly as possible. Defer tours, elective conversations, and unpacking until you enter your active stage.

49. Forget the past.

Begin immediately to live in your new time zone, if you haven't already changed over. Experts counsel that you should avoid gradual adaptation at this point, even if it means shocking your system into accepting your destination time. Social cues—external zeitgebers from the world around you—become even more influential once you've reached your destination. Since much of your body's adjustment depends on your mental adjustment, nothing's gained by allowing your mind to creep back home every time you look at a clock.

50. Go to bed and arise when the natives do.

If you've booked your arrival close to bedtime at your destination, you're apt to have an easier time falling asleep, regardless of your travel direction, since you will have less than a full waking day to endure. If you have flown east and haven't yet adapted to DT, you're likely to experience wakefulness when you need to be sleeping. While you can't will yourself to fall asleep, it's still critical that your body experience the zeitgeber of preparing for and getting to bed on DT.

If you have flown west of your point of origin, until your body clocks are fully adjusted you will probably awaken anywhere from one to many hours before your hosts, depending on the number of time zones traveled. If you do, force yourself to stay in bed. While sleeping (wearing a dark eyeshade helps) is preferable, even resting will help reset your clock. Don't arise and get active until you would normally on DT.

Light Strategies at Your Destination

First Day After Arrival
• Live on the light-dark schedule of destination time (DT).

Eastbound: Get outside in early morning daylight for an hour or two, and avoid bright light in late afternoon.

Westbound: Avoid early morning light, but be certain to get light exposure in late afternoon.

• *If your pretrip schedule precluded starting light-dark adjustments earlier than your travel day,* follow the advice of circadian research pioneer Alfred J. Lewy and his abbreviated adjustment program:

Eastbound: In the first few days at your

destination, when you are trying to advance your clock by doing everything earlier, seek bright morning sun in the first few hours of daylight. If you have crossed *six or fewer* zones, avoid bright light in the afternoon. If you have crossed *six or more* zones, seek bright light at midday and avoid light in the morning.

Westbound: If you have crossed *six or fewer* zones, seek late afternoon sun to delay your clock, and avoid it in the morning. If you have crossed *six or more* zones, seek strong midday light, and avoid bright morning light.[2]

51. Don't isolate yourself.

Studies show that solitary travelers who keep to themselves (and to their rooms) once they arrive adjust much more slowly to a new time zone than those traveling in groups, or with a companion, or those who are quick to explore the local scene. "You can't begin to sop up social and temporal cues in isolation," explains author Donald Kowet in *The Jet Lag Book*. "You need to seek social stimuli." So, especially if you are traveling by yourself, go out of your way the first few days to seek company and mental stimulation away from your hotel room.

[2]Hauri, Peter, Ph.D., and Shirley Linde, Ph.D. *No More Sleepless Nights* (New York: John Wiley, 1990).

Food Strategies at Your Destination

First Day After Arrival

- According to the Ehret diet, *meals and meal patterns should be aligned with those that are normal to destination time.* He advises eating proteins when you need energy and carbohydrates when you need to sleep.

- Wurtman's recommendations: *Make food work for you.* If you have flown west—from the East Coast to Hawaii, for instance—to get on the Hawaiian schedule, eat a high-carbohydrate breakfast. Since you'll probably awaken early, such a meal will help delay your tendency to rev up too early. Try to sleep as late as you can and don't give in to food cravings, even though you will awaken hungry in such an instance (since it's already lunchtime in your home time [HT]). Don't consume caffeinated substances before 8 A.M. DT.

- If you are ravenous between meals, *nibble on crackers* or a piece of fruit, but don't eat a real meal until lunch.

- Lunchtime in your new destination may coincide with dinnertime at home, so *fight the impulse to eat huge portions,* which will just leave you drowsy—the opposite of what you want to happen—while your body tries to digest the food.

- *Eat foods that do not prompt the manufacture or release of calming or alertness chemicals.* Such foods include clear soups, fruit, nonstarchy vegetables, a chef's salad without the dressing or mayonnaise—in fact, many of the same ingredients you have eaten on the Ehret diet's fast days. Your meals should contain no fats, no alcohol, and only unsweetened fruit for dessert.
- In afternoons at your destination, if it is close to your HT bedtime, *at first you will probably have a hard time staying awake.* Coffee or tea at these times is a good foil. Or take a short (less than an hour) nap. Follow your slumber with fifteen to twenty minutes of exercise, a brisk walk, or a swim, which will help boost your metabolism and body temperature—marks of alertness.
- *If you have flown west, delay your evening meals as long as possible the first several days.* Then eat high-protein, low-fat, low-carbohydrate foods that are easy to digest, and consume no alcohol. Coffee or tea at the end of a meal is permissible, since either should help you stay awake until normal DT bedtime.

Activity Strategies at Your Destination

First Day After Arrival
Eastbound: Plan rigorous activities to co-incide with the early morning sunlight and restful activities for late afternoon (a time to avoid bright light).

Westbound: Plan a restful morning and follow it with an active afternoon.

- **Abbreviated adjustment program:** If your pretrip schedule did not allow you to start adjusting your sleep/wake cycle until your travel day, then follow these tips:

Eastbound: In the first few days at your destination, as you are trying to advance your clock, be vigorously active in the first few hours of daylight. If you have crossed *six or fewer* zones, schedule more restful activities in late afternoon. If you have crossed *six or more* zones, engage in lively activity at midday, after a restful morning.

Westbound: If you have crossed *six or fewer* zones, engage in late afternoon activity (outdoors, if possible)—to help delay body clocks—but rest in the morning. If you have crossed *six or more* zones, be active in midday light after resting in the morning.

- If you suspect you're supposed to be active but feel too groggy to remember, choose activity over immobility.

Light Strategies at Your Destination

Second Day After Arrival

Live on local time, seeking intense sunlight or dark at the same times you did the day you landed (see page 103).

Food Strategies at Your Destination

Second Day After Arrival

As you acclimate to living on local time, use foods to support your sleep-wake schedule. If you need to be awake and active but find your energy flagging between meals, eat a sweet carbohydrate snack for a quick energy boost. Caffeine also may be a help at this time. (But limit your carbohydrates to snack time: proteins are still best at mealtimes when you need to be awake for a long period.)

If you find yourself unable to sleep or if you awaken in the middle of the night, try a piece of candy or other small sweetened snack to get the serotonin level up. Remember to stay away from a heavy protein meal at night, favoring carbohydrates instead. Avoid fats. If you have a meal that contains both carbohydrate and protein, be sure to eat the carbohydrate first if you are trying to induce sleep.

Activity Strategies at Your Destination

Second Day After Arrival

Live on local time, exaggerating activity and rest efforts to give your body stronger time cues while resetting body clocks. In other words, don't just walk; speed walk or run. And don't simply lie down with your clothes on in a room bathed with light; change into sleeping clothes, pull shades or curtains, and climb into bed. You may feel fatigued owing to the strains of travel, but keeping active and resting only at the appropriate times will help you maintain your new sleep-wake schedule.

Light Strategies at Your Destination

Third Day After Arrival

Maintain your light-exposure/light-avoidance schedule (see page 103, Lewy's abbreviated adjustment schedule), seeking sunlight or dark to reinforce your new schedule. Continue to use this reinforcement device until you feel fully acclimated.

Activity Strategies at Your Destination

Third Day After Arrival

Same strategies as day two.

52. Use rituals.

Rituals—activities we do routinely that mark events or schedules—provide strong social cues to sleeping and waking. While the body needs three to four weeks to settle fully into a new routine, according to Hauri, reinstituting familiar rituals or daily habits from home can speed your adjustment.

- **To induce sleep:** Replicate your presleep rituals from home: take a short walk (if that's what you do normally before bed), brush your teeth, wash your face, and spend the last hour before bed quietly—all familiar signals to your body that you are preparing for sleep. Also incorporate these habits, known as good *sleep hygiene*:
  Make your bedroom as dark and noise-free as you can. Avoid caffeine and anything more than light alcohol use. Don't go to bed full (or starving). If you smoke, try to avoid smoking for several hours before bed. With the help of an alarm clock, arise at the same time each day. Follow regular mealtimes, if possible.
- **To promote wakefulness**: Practice good sleep hygiene, such as regular bed- and waking times, to give yourself time cues and establish a familiar schedule. When you awaken, engage in the same waking rituals you use at home, such as bathing, washing your face, brushing your teeth, having a morning cup of coffee, and reading the paper. If you find your energy and alertness flagging during the day, import a ritual from home

to revive yourself: a late afternoon cold drink or coffee, a splash of water on your face, your regular midday jog or brisk walk, preferably in sunlight.

53. Let food work for you.

Remember that proteins perk and carbos crash. You'll want to apply the same food principles you've used since you began your anti–jet lag adaptation (examples of high-protein and high-carbohydrate foods appear in appendix A). Timing of meals is important: it's never good to try to sleep immediately after a meal. Sleep experts generally advise at least a four-hour gap between dinner or supper and bedtime. If you anticipate trouble falling asleep, eat a light snack high in carbohydrates one to two hours before bed. Conversely, if it's not anywhere near bedtime and you still can't keep your eyes open, eat energizing snacks that are higher in protein than carbohydrates but low in fat (a low-fat granola bar, for example). Carbohydrates will give you a short-term boost, while the slower-acting proteins will kick in to give you longer-lasting stamina.

Endocrinologist and author Judith Wurtman, Ph.D., advises that small snacks every several hours will keep your digestive system working, which in turn will keep you awake. Don't overdo the calories: when snacking or eating meals to initiate sleep or promote alertness, you need only a little carbohydrate or protein to set the appropriate brain chemicals to work.

54. Try essential oils to help you get past jet lag symptoms.

Essential oils of chamomile, geranium, and lavender added to your bathwater are thought by aromatherapists to help induce restful sleep. Author Jude Brown, *Aromatherapy for Travelers* (Thorsens 1995), recommends chamomile, geranium, and lavender oils, in concentrations of one drop each mixed with a 2.4 ml base oil for your trip, for best effects. For those who need to plunge right into full schedules upon arrival, she recommends a different combination for "an uplifting effect" on the senses that results in a wide-awake state: 2 drops eucalyptus oil, 1 drop geranium oil, and 3 drops rosemary oil in a 2.5 ml. base oil. Also use this mixture in mornings on your trip, or use it in the shower as a last rinse (it does not cleanse) by applying it with a sponge. She recommends following each bath while traveling with this aromatic body rub, to sooth the nerves and relax the mind and body: 2 drops each of geranium and lavender oil, mixed in a 20 ml base oil. Essential and base oil preparations can be purchased in health food stores or aromatherapy boutiques.

55. Try ginseng to restore your endurance.

"Siberian ginseng is excellent for relieving jet lag symptoms," writes naturopathic physician

Steven Schechter in the July/August 1995 *Natural Health*. For the first few days following your flight, the dosage he recommends is one teaspoon three times a day, on an empty stomach to help absorption.

This natural substance, said to prolong life and cure many ills, has been used by various civilizations for more than two thousand years. Siberian ginseng (*Eleutherococcus senticosus*) is an adaptogen, which is a substance that protects against mental and physical stress. As such, it is reputed to help disrupted body functions return to normal more quickly than they would otherwise, resulting in improved physical endurance.

If using ginseng appeals to you, be sure to check with your doctor first. You should know that the efficacy of Siberian ginseng is controversial, since some believe it has little or no effect. Even though the Food and Drug Administration rates it as a safe herbal, an herbal is a drug: it can interact with other medications you may be taking.

56. Try a cup of passionflower or valerian tea.

Passionflower and valerian are two herbal remedies used to induce sleep and are often used to treat jet lag symptoms. For a mildly tranquilizing herbal sleep remedy, passionflower—generally available from health food stores—is brewed into a tea using one teaspoon of tincture in a cup of boiling water, one hour before bedtime, then followed with a second dose fifteen minutes before bedtime. Passionflower is an ingredient in a number of sedative-hypnotic drugs sold in Europe, according to pharmacognosist Varro Tyler, Ph.D.[3]

Valerian is also widely used in Europe to promote sleep and sleep quality, and it is used similarly in the United States. Valerian's odor, which many find unpleasant, is a deterrent to its widespread use, even though the herb's efficacy as a sedative is documented. You may want to try the more palatable capsule form, rather than tea. Remember: Treat passionflower and valerian and all herbs as you would any other medicine you use.

57. Get your daily dose of B-complex vitamins.

A shortage of B-complex vitamins contributes to fatigue, the last thing you need when your residual jet lag is begging you to hit the sack. Furthermore, a Japanese study, conducted at Hokkaido University School of Medicine in Sapporo, indicated that one B-complex vitamin in particular, B_{12}, may also help in phase advancing your body clocks—in other words, resetting them forward, as when you've flown east.[4] It apparently does this by increasing light sensitivity of the circadian clock.

[3]Clare Kowalchick, and William H. Hylton, eds. *Rodale's Illustrated Encyclopedia of Herbs* (Emmaus, Penn.: Rodale Press, 1987).
[4]*Experientia* (August 15, 1992).

Those who eat regular, nutritious meals may be getting all of the B-complex vitamins they need. (If not, see chapter 2 for a discussion of minimum dietary requirements.) For treating insomnia, David S. Bell, M.D., author of *Curing Fatigue*, recommends increasing B_{12} intake to 50–100 mg daily, taken in two doses with meals.[5] Foods rich in vitamin B_{12} include liver and organ meats, muscle meats, fish, eggs, shellfish, and milk and most dairy products, except butter. Be aware that B-complex vitamins can affect some people differently, causing them to be energized rather than sedated. For this reason, it's a good idea to discuss your vitamin program with your physician and test your B_{12} reaction before you take your trip.

58. Don't nap.

Whether you've traveled east or west, you're going to hit a time of day when your body craves a nap. Experts agree that naps are not helpful for—and may even harm—your jet lag adjustment progress. Your body may try to trick you into napping by making you crave sedating carbohydrates, explains Wurtman, a food urge you must resist if you want to stay awake. If it's a matter of collapsing unless you have a nap, make sure it's less than an hour, says Robert Giller, M.D., author of *Natural Prescriptions*.

[5]Emmaus, Penn.: Rodale Press, 1993.

59. Exercise away that jet lag.

"The first thing you should try to do when you get to your destination is exercise to loosen up your legs after long hours of sitting in a cramped seat," recommends Timothy Moore, Ph.D., in the October 1994 *Women's Sports and Fitness*. Moore, director of program development at the National Hospital for Orthopedics and Rehabilitation, says that thirty minutes on a stationary bike is a good exercise choice because it offers "light tension and high rpms, both of which stretch without taxing your tired muscles." Moore also recommends water exercise for its soothing effects. Don't do anything that works the muscles hard against much resistance, he warns the newly landed traveler. So, just plan on swimming or walking—and leave the weights in your suitcase.

Jet Lag Book author Kowet concurs that exercise is important the first day, but recommends not diving into a heavy schedule of workouts if you aren't used to it. Begin with standard relaxation exercises such as deep breathing and progressive muscle relaxation. Kowet recommends jumping rope as a travel exercise without peer: a fifteen-minute jump is equivalent to running one mile.

A word of caution, though: If, when you get to your destination, you are supposed to be in a resting-dark period, table all exercise until you enter your active-waking period. Otherwise you'll undo your anti–jet lag efforts.

60. Use exercise to help you sleep.

When your body temperature starts falling—a
normal nighttime occurrence—you get sleepy, less
alert, and less active. Strenuous activity raises
your temperature and wakes you, which is why we
have advised you not to exercise too close to bedtime. Your sleeping temperature is lower than
your daytime—or core—temperature, and it drops
to its lowest point during your deepest sleep,
which for normal sleepers is somewhere between
2 A.M. and 4 A.M. (the same time as your switchpoint, discussed in chapter 1). Doing twenty
minutes of aerobic exercise—enough to raise your
normal temperature by two degrees—will influence your body temperature to drop five to six
hours after your exercise ends. If jet lag hangover
is interfering with your sleep, by exercising five to
six hours before your bedtime, you can engineer
the time you want to fall asleep.

61. If you're using drug therapy, stop as soon as you can.

Even though they clear most adults' bodies in
three to five hours, short-acting hypnotics—sleeping pills—are not intended for prolonged use. For
the jet-lagged traveler, sleeping pills (*only* the
short-acting variety) should be used to promote
rest on a long flight of six or more hours and/or to
sleep the first couple of nights at the destination
as acclimatization continues. Among their other
properties, most short-acting sleeping pills alter

or eliminate the REM (rapid eye movement) stage of your sleep; REM is the stage of the deepest sleep that is most restorative to your physical and mental states. Thus, taken longer than needed, short-acting hypnotics won't lead to better sleep; they will prevent it.

62. Stay away from the local culinary delicacies.

New places and customs can tempt travelers to eat local foods with abandon as soon as they've unpacked. If you've just flown to another country where the diet may differ significantly from yours, give your stomach—and the rest of your jet lag–challenged body—a break. Until you feel more like your usual self, avoid rich foods and sauces, highly spiced or salted foods, and fried delicacies. It's also prudent to eat lighter meals than you would normally so that your digestive system can work on resetting its clock, rather than on digesting the deep-fried pigeon you just ate for breakfast.

Preparing for the Return Trip

What you experienced after flying in one direction, says Bell in *Chronic Fatigue,* will be different from what you feel after flying the other way. So when you head home after a trip of five days or more, is it advisable to try to beat jet lag going the other way? The answer is yes. What and how you choose to do it will hinge on these pertinent factors:

- **how many time zones you've crossed.** At three or fewer, especially if you'll be westbound flying home, you may elect to ignore the resultant jet lag, which should be minor, and do nothing but enjoy the last few days of your travel.
- **whether you'll be flying east or west.** Those flying east back to their point of origin should have more concerns owing to the more difficult time adjustment.
- **how hard jet lag hit you on the outbound leg of your trip.** If it knocked you for a loop, you will want to undertake some anti–jet lag measures before setting out for home; regardless of the intrusiveness of these efforts on your last days of travel.
- **length of your trip.** If it's been relatively short, for example, you have traveled west across nine time zones to stay for only a week, you will barely have time to attend to activities at your destination before preparing for the trip back. So, you probably won't have time to revive your anti–jet lag maneuvers. A longer trip, on the other hand, may allow you time to prepare both ways.
- **your schedule.** If your trip across six time zones is ten days long, but you have meetings, tours, or other events heavily scheduled through the last day before you travel, it's an easy bet

that you'll not be able to engage in a full anti–jet lag effort as you did in your pretrip phase.

Here are the several principal options open to you for beating jet lag on the return leg of your journey:

Option 1. Go with the flow and don't take steps to fight homeward-bound jet lag.

If you elect this option, you may want to factor in a day or two of downtime at home to recuperate from the jet lag effects you are going to suffer, regardless of which direction you travel home. Business, government agencies, and commercial airlines are increasingly trying to build in one or more days of recuperative time for their employees who do transmeridian travel. Try to schedule a return flight that lands as close to your normal bedtime (home time) as possible.

Option 2. Fight jet lag on the home front by taking steps while you're traveling.

If you'd rather fight jet lag on both fronts, and the length of your trip allows it, fully reverse the strategy you followed when you flew to your destination.

Let's say you crossed six time zones flying west to your ten-day vacation spot. You started your acclimatization program four days before you flew, leaving you to finish adjusting on day one of your trip (travel day) and the day following. If you were to fully adjust by the day after your return flight, you would have three days (days three, four, and five) of freedom from jet lag concerns before having to reverse engines and begin preparing for your homeward flight east (day six through the day following your travel day).

If you're one of the people jet lag typically clobbers, you may decide that cramping your regular eating and meeting styles on vacation or business—that is, if your schedule permits—in order to do the whole program in reverse is well worth the effort. Only you know. You should also be influenced if you are flying east (the more difficult of the adjustments) or if you have a schedule of back-to-back important activities at home.

If you have taken a longer trip—for example, one that lasts from two weeks to several months—reversing the whole program to avoid jet lag once you get home is the logical choice. Begin the same number of days in advance of your return that you did when you started your pretrip preparation. (If you are returning to the west, you might cut a day or two off of your efforts without many noticeable effects.) Once home, continue the program until your jet lag symptoms have disappeared.

Option 3. An amalgam of #1 and #2.

For a trip of a week to ten days, a compromise option may appeal, since you can start resetting your body clocks before you arrive home, but the regimen will cut only briefly into your vacation or business activities and menus. You may not have time (or interest) to do the same level of advance work as you did before your trip, but even getting a day or two of adjustment under your belt before you board your return flight will help offset jet lag effects on the trip home and thereafter.

For the ten-day trip we discussed in #2, you might begin your program only one or two days before you travel, rather than the three to four you followed on your pretrip plan. Thus, when you land back at your point of origin, your circadian clock will be one-third rather than two-thirds reset (so plan to undergo another three to four days of disruption before you're fully back to normal).

Your best bet, should you choose this option, is to schedule a day (or weekend) of downtime once you get home so that you can reduce your travel-related stress and jet lag symptoms as much as possible before you resume your full spate of activities. If you have the luxury of a day or two off once you've landed, don't spend the whole time sleeping: be fastidious about following your food, light, and activity strategies.

You may have noticed that we have not addressed transmeridian travel lasting less than a week. We do cover such shorter travel—very typical for business trips or personal emergencies—in our frequent flyer box in chapter 2.

You now have comprehensive *natural* tips for arresting jet lag's effects. But the question still remains—will there ever be a cure that prevents jet lag altogether or at least cuts its duration? Chron-obiological research is making advances toward just such a resolution. In chapter 5 we take a look at what's on the horizon.

CHAPTER 5

The Promise
of Research

While research shows that sleeping pills and anti–jet lag diets can reduce the symptoms of jet lag symptoms effectively, are light therapy and melatonin supplementation likely to figure into the ultimate cure for jet lag? Circadian research projects centering on light and melatonin are now in progress throughout the international community. With each study, more is learned about the body's timekeepers and their mechanisms for setting, maintaining, and resetting circadian rhythms.

Light Therapy Status and Developments

In chapter 1 we described the physiological processes involved in setting circadian rhythms. New research has further defined the interaction of light and melatonin. A decade ago scientists suspected that the brain's suprachiasmic nuclei (SCN) had another role besides that of the body's principal circadian pacemaker. Since then, studies have unraveled increasingly more detail on the intricate process of circadian pacesetting. Research teams have identified a direct link between the eyes and the brain: when retinas register light, they then send impulses along an optic pathway to the brain's SCN, which in turn signals the pineal gland to stop production and secretion of melatonin.

Studies have been able definitively to link sleep-onset brain chemicals such as melatonin with other neurotransmitters that function when the body is awake. At the point that melatonin secretion ceases, the arousal hormones—cortisol and epinephrine—initiate waking responses that include raising body temperature and increasing alertness. Later in the day, natural light dims and darkness sets in. The cessation of light impulses cues melatonin production, which lowers body temperature and energy levels, preparing the body for sleep. The flow of melatonin into the bloodstream continues for a total of twelve hours—peaking at 2 A.M. or 3 A.M.—then stops as the retinas once again register daylight.

Chronobiologists have long known that circadian rhythms are set by light cues of sunrise, dusk, and even the onset of different seasons. Once these patterns have been established—or entrained—they are maintained, even when an organism is immersed in total darkness. What has not been known until the last decade is what triggers internal clocks to go out of sequence with their external cues—as they do in jet lag—and how to reset them when they do. More and more, research findings point to light—not only as the essential component of circadian timing, but also as the clock's reset button. Recent studies have established the predictability of the body's reaction to light and melatonin (called the *phase-response curve*), and we now know how to manipulate the body's clock through scheduled light exposure.

Significant Discoveries about Light

Of the many current studies on light and circadian rhythm, the following findings—each of which has implications for jet lag—are notable:

- *In 1996 research identified a complex daily genetic protein regeneration and disintegration process,* cued by natural light cycles, that resets the body's clocks. The studies, conducted independently by four different U.S. research teams, show that introduction of light pulses destroys these proteins or blocks the regeneration process, throwing body clocks off. With this understanding of how light functions as a master switch and how basic genetic mechanisms react with light, scientists believe they can develop drugs that will mimic or mask the effects of light to solve jet lag and other circadian disorders.

• *Light need not be bright,* as had previously been thought, nor must it be full-spectrum light (such as natural daylight) to close down melatonin production. While brighter light may drop melatonin levels lower, new studies indicate that even dim light can negatively affect melatonin secretion. Some studies have shown that low levels of indoor light, which is seldom full-spectrum or even as intense as daylight on a cloudy day, can alter circadian rhythm. This is particularly significant for those following light therapy for their jet lag: it illustrates why total darkness is so vital during resting periods.

• *The retinas are critical to establishing a regular pattern and maintaining circadian rhythms,* whether a person is sighted or blind. Studies reported in 1995 by Boston researchers show that the human eye has two functions, only one of which—conscious vision—is to see. It also independently registers the light impulses that travel through a tract in the optic nerve to regulate the body's clock. This suggests that some blind people can have a normal hormonal response to light. A 1996 animal study suggests that in addition to registering light impulses to prompt the secretion of melatonin elsewhere, retinas may even contain their own timepieces that produce their own melatonin.

• *Current research targets the molecular level and fundamental makeup of the retina, SCN, and hypothalamus region of the brain.* New studies seem to show that fibrous proteins in the hypothalamus may be providing an important route through which stimuli other than light can affect the SCN, the body's key pacemaker. The finding holds promise for developing a medicine to augment time-setting signals along this route.

Light Therapy: What's Available

Already on the market for light therapy are light boxes, usually containing up to 10,000 lux of fluorescent lighting; light visors that direct light into the eyes (though they don't interfere with reading), worn at prescribed times during and after travel; a transmeridian schedule that uses light exposure to manipulate secretion of melatonin, developed in 1995 by National Institute of Mental Health circadian researchers led by Dan

A. Oren, M.D. (described under the special light strategies throughout this book); and a lighted "globe" cued by an alarm clock that gradually becomes brighter to simulate daybreak and daylight (see appendix B).

Numerous light-related therapies to regulate circadian rhythm, anti–jet lag devices, and drugs are now under study and/or imminently bound for the U.S. market. They include the following:

- **artificial light sources** in the form of hats, visors, and light boxes that are more flexible and portable than their predecessors (some are available now—see appendix B).
- **dark glasses, contact lenses, and low-density lighting** with a partial-spectrum light block that will allow the user to register only those spectra of light known not to affect melatonin production (patent granted and now in development).
- **a mechanism and process that stimulate the same response that light does to reset circadian rhythms**.
- **A "jet lag pill"** that would immediately reset the circadian clock upon landing in a new time zone. University of Bath circadian researchers conjectured in *Chronobiology International* (1994) that such a drug might act by affecting the body's signals that regulate the internal clocks, affecting the body's clock directly, or affecting the links between the body's clocks. Each

involves complexities that will require a better knowledge of the work of neurotransmitters.

Melatonin Therapy Status and Developments

The success of treatment for jet lag by appropriately timed exposure to bright light, according to circadian research pioneer Alfred J. Lewy, M.D., Ph.D., can be achieved equally well by appropriately timed melatonin administration.

Since it was first isolated as a hormone in 1958, melatonin studies have spanned almost four decades. Yet this substance has recently catapulted into the headlines, hailed as the safe and natural cure-all for everything from cancer and aging to contraception and sleep disorders, including jet lag. Jet lag, in fact, is what made melatonin the household word of the decade. An April 1994 *Condé Nast Traveler* article proclaimed: "Jet lag's familiar symptoms . . . were markedly alleviated by taking supplemental [synthetic] melatonin capsules." The report was based on a 1986 British double-blind study showing that melatonin reduced eastbound jet lag by as much as 40 percent and westbound by up to 60 percent, with minimal to no side effects reported.

Other, newer studies have consistently supported the British data and demonstrated melatonin's effectiveness. Yet melatonin therapy is controversial in the medical community for several reasons:

• *Melatonin is considered a food supplement, not a drug, in the United States. As such, the strength and purity of melatonin supplements are not overseen by any regulatory body.* Critics are quick to point to the tryptophan scare of 1989, when an impure batch of the synthesized amino acid (since then withdrawn from the market) reached consumers and caused a rare and irreversible muscle disease in more than one thousand U.S. users. Foes of regulation, on the other hand, note that melatonin has been taken for years by persons studying and participating in various sleep and jet lag studies, without adverse side effects. In addition, no one has ever died of a megadose of the substance, they say.

Melatonin itself isn't likely to be classified as a drug anytime soon for two reasons: 1) more stringent clinical studies on its efficacy have yet to be conducted, say members of the medical and scientific communities; and 2) under current U.S. law, natural substances cannot be patented. The latter means that any company can market a melatonin formula that has been researched and developed by another. Because this limits profitability, no private-sector funds are available for unpatentable substances. Moreover, federal research funds have been drying up. Instead, drug companies are trying to come up with patentable melatonin analogs that share some of the qualities but have a different molecular structure than melatonin. In 1995 more than one hundred had been patented and many, many more compounds have been created that simulate some aspect of melatonin.

- *Researchers and medical practitioners alike worry about the current sources of unregulated melatonin.* Most strongly favor limiting supplements to the synthetic variety, created in laboratories from pharmaceutical-grade raw materials. The natural form, also available, comes from the pineal glands of cows, causing worry about the possibility of contracting a bovine disease called *scrapie*. Since 1996, when Britain experienced "mad-cow disease," a fatal neurological illness related to scrapie that is passed on to humans from cows, the concern over natural forms of melatonin has intensified.

- *Wrong timing of melatonin supplementation can create the opposite effect of what is desired.* A study led by Lewy, reported in the October 1992 *Chronobiology International*, showed that melatonin shifts circadian rhythm according to the time of day it is taken: if taken in the morning, melatonin delays circadian rhythm and allows the user to sleep later. If taken in the afternoon or early evening, it advances the body clock, permitting the user to sleep earlier. Users who don't understand this phase-response curve can worsen their jet lag.

- *It remains to be seen whether taking melatonin will cause long-term side effects.* However, the consensus to date, based on empirical and anecdotal data, seems to be that side effects from melatonin for jet lag are negligible and not adverse *when the substance is taken in small doses*.

Josephine Arendt, Ph.D., who conducted the first broad-based jet lag study of melatonin in 1983, has collected data on melatonin supplementation's side effects since 1981. Her data show that minor short-term side effects that have appeared in extremely low percentages among study volunteers include mild daytime sleepiness (8.9 percent), occasional mental impairment such as "fuzziness" or giddiness (2.9 percent), headache (2.9 percent), and nausea (0.9 percent). Dry mouth and accelerated heartbeat are mentioned less often. Taken in much larger doses than are currently recommended for jet lag treatment, melatonin can act as a mild contraceptive in women. A series of 1994 studies showed that melatonin produces far fewer negative memory and performance effects than do the short-acting benzodiazepines that are in use to offset jet lag fatigue. In spite of the good news, a number of considerations about melatonin as a jet-lag therapy need to be settled:

• *Additional broad-based and rigorous clinical trials on melatonin need to be performed or completed,* argue many members of the medical and scientific communities, who feel the current body of melatonin knowledge has been gained principally from limited, small-group studies. Those in disagreement cite findings from more than one hundred published placebo-controlled studies and point to a range of study sizes—from 10 to more than 1,400 volunteers—centered at some of the world's preeminent research institutions.

- *More research is needed concerning appropriate melatonin dosages.* Until 1996 melatonin was marketed in pill and capsule forms ranging from 1 to 2 mg. Concurrently with this, researchers were concluding that as little as 0.1 to 0.5 mg (roughly equal to a few grains of salt) might be the best dosage since it most closely resembles the tiny amount of melatonin found naturally in the body. Richard J. Wurtman, M.D., Ph.D., one of the world's foremost melatonin researchers, told *The Wall Street Journal* in 1996 that he feared too high a dose of melatonin would induce "round-the-clock drowsiness, hypothermia, loss of infection-fighting power, and a rise in the hormone prolactin." Recently, capsules containing only 200 mcg—0.2 mg—of synthetic melatonin as well as timed-release capsules have reached the U.S. market (but they still lack regulation). Even more attention will be focused on melatonin supplementation dosage if, as some studies suggest, the retina is found to produce melatonin, say doctors and researchers, lest an overdose permanently damage the retina.

- *Many members of the medical and scientific communities are openly appalled at the bandwagon effect surrounding melatonin.* Physicians and scientists alike denounce as dangerous the widespread claims that melatonin is the world's miracle cure-all. Natural medicine enthusiast Andrew Weil, M.D., summed up the feelings of many doctors and researchers when he told *New Age Journal* (February 1996) that he felt uneasy about recommending melatonin as a daily tonic. "Because it's a brain hormone, it is certain to have general effects on many systems of the body, and we may not know what all of its actions actually are."

Melatonin Therapies: What's Available?

If you elect to try melatonin supplements for jet lag, seek advice from your doctor and start with the very smallest dosage possible. To take the recommended 0.1 to 0.5 mg, using the new 200 mcg capsule will be most convenient; otherwise plan on breaking even the next size into several pieces. Many researchers strongly discourage melatonin supplementation by patients they consider high-risk until more is known about melatonin's overall effects. Pioneering melatonin researcher Russel J. Reiter, Ph.D., includes those persons taking steroids; women who are pregnant, wanting to conceive, or lactating; those suffering from depression or mental illness, allergies, autoimmune diseases, or immune system cancers; and children.

Suggestions by researchers of how much and when to take melatonin vary widely.

Timing Breakthroughs

An important 1992 study, headed by Lewy, demonstrated that melatonin's phase-response curve (PRC)—a person's switchpoint, when melatonin administration stops advancing and begins delaying the circadian clock—falls at a time directly opposite the PRC and switchpoint of light exposure. Thus, the study showed that melatonin taken in the afternoon or evening "simulates the sunset" and advances the clock (versus advancing with early morning bright light), while morning melatonin therapy "delays the dawn" (versus delaying with late afternoon light exposure). These findings have helped researchers begin to pinpoint the most effective melatonin supplementation patterns, although there are still variations in timing of melatonin therapy.

Before, during, and after travel therapy generally follows researcher Lewy's findings. To cut jet lag by up to 50 percent, Lewy suggests that a traveler should take one 0.5 mg pill the day before travel (eastbound, early afternoon; westbound, at wakeup time), one on the travel day at the same time, and one on the arrival day (at the destination time equivalent to when it had been taken the previous two days).[1] Each day's administration of

[1] *The New York Times* (September 27, 1995).

melatonin shifts the clock by about two hours, he says; thus, for longer trips extend the therapy for another several days.

Following a different approach, Arendt advises her westbound travelers *not* to take melatonin in the early morning on the day of travel because it induces too much drowsiness. Instead she recommends that the westbound traveler take one 5 mg pill each night at bedtime on the four nights following the flight. For the eastbound traveler, she suggests one 5 mg pill taken in late afternoons for one to two days before traveling, then another at bedtime for the four nights following the flight.

These two vastly different applications of melatonin supplementation—each producing positive results—are markedly different from a well-publicized 1993 New Zealand study of an international jet crew. In that study those who took 5 mg during and after the flight regained energy, good mood, and alertness faster than the crews who began the supplementation pretravel. Surprisingly, this latter group experienced *even worse* jet lag than study participants who had taken nothing at all.

Researchers hypothesize that melatonin may work best in those who normally have a stable sleep-wake cycle, but not in such travelers as airline crews, whose cycles are chronically disturbed. Also, since the melatonin/PRC-timing relationship was unknown at the time of the study, it is possible, say researchers, that some participants may have taken melatonin at the wrong time of day, thus extending rather than shortening jet lag.

While scientists continue to refine their knowledge about synthetic melatonin therapy, you can take steps to preserve and promote the amount of natural melatonin in your body. Here's how:

- **Recognize that any of these activities depletes your melatonin supply**: sleeping with the lights on; taking ibuprofen or aspirin; taking beta-blockers such as propranolol (Inderal), atenolol (Tenormin), or metoprolol (Lopressor, Toprol); taking calcium channel blockers or some other antihypertensive medicines, which may have less of an inhibitory effect if taken earlier in the day; taking such antidepressants in the benzodiazepine family as diazepam (Valium) and alprazolam (Xanax); and taking vitamin B_{12} supplements in large quantities (not the amount found in multivitamins). In addition, caffeine, tobacco, and alcohol have all been shown to lessen the amount of natural melatonin in the system. External factors affecting human melatonin levels are still under study. For instance, researchers continue to look for a link between melatonin levels and electromagnetic fields, such as those created by power lines or household wiring and microwave ovens, electric blankets, telephones, and the like.
- **Help preserve your natural melatonin supply** by increasing your exposure to natural daylight (an hour a day at 1,000 lux or more). Take

a regular light break outdoors, wear UV-protective sunglasses light enough to let light enter your eyes, and add light sources in your office or home—including painting walls light, reflective colors. Minimize exposure to bright light at night by putting dimmers on lights. Read by lower light at night and turn lights off while watching TV. Wear a sleep mask if your partner reads in bed while you are trying to sleep, and use a night-light if you have to get up at night. Also, get more sleep, which enhances melatonin production.

- **Eat melatonin-friendly foods.** Fescue, a grass that is high in melatonin, can be found in tonic juices sold at juice bars and in some health food stores. If you're more conventional, eat oats, sweet corn, rice, ginger, tomatoes, bananas, barley; toasted or cooked oatmeal, oat granola; rice cakes, noodles, or cereals; and cornbread muffins or flakes. If you are trying to influence sleep, try these in snacks an hour before bedtime.

Since the pineal gland synthesizes melatonin by converting tryptophan to serotonin and then to melatonin, eating foods rich in tryptophan can increase melatonin. But be sure to accompany or precede tryptophan-rich foods with carbohydrates that will help boost the tryptophan into the brain. Try turkey, milk and soy products, pumpkin seeds, chicken, watermelon seeds, almonds, peanuts, or brewer's yeast as tryptophan sources.

- **Be sure these melatonin-boosting vitamins and minerals are in your diet,** recommends health writer Nathaniel Mead in *Natural Health* magazine:

   Vitamin B$_3$ (niacin), 100 mg daily. Your body uses B$_3$ to convert tryptophan to serotonin and melatonin, so add to your natural reserves through supplementation, or before bed have a B$_3$-rich snack, containing such ingredients as dried apricots, barley, beef liver, brewer's yeast, chicken, halibut, peanuts, pork, salmon, sunflower seeds, swordfish, tuna, turkey, veal, and wheat bran.

   Vitamin B$_6$ (pyridoxine), 25–50 mg. Taken daily in the morning, B$_6$ may stimulate melatonin production. Foods high in B$_6$ include avocados, bananas, brewer's yeast, carrots, lentils, rice, salmon, shrimp, soybeans, tuna, wheat bran, wheat germ, whole-wheat flour, and many enriched breakfast cereals.

   Also, get adequate **calcium** (1,200 mg daily) and **magnesium** (500 mg daily), but, as with any vitamin or mineral regimen, don't megadose.

While it's exciting to know that safe and approved comprehensive and totally effective jet lag solutions are right around the corner, safely defeating jet lag is already possible if you are using the variety of natural approaches we've described for you. Use the combination of tips that work best for you, and you will find that the aftermath of flying across many time zones is no longer the ordeal it used to be. *Bon voyage!*

Foods to Help You Beat Jet Lag

Avoid fatty foods, including chocolate and anything fried or sautéed, which are difficult to digest and interfere with sleep. Foods highlighted in bold type are classes of foods; others are examples of snacks you may wish to carry in-flight or eat during a stopover.

Alertness-Producing Foods

Best: High-Protein

These may include a carbohydrate component, but in smaller proportions than protein. If eating a carbohydrate/protein combination, start with protein to allow the brain to block serotonin release.

almonds
beans of all kinds (try to avoid while airborne)
beef, jerky
beef, lean roast (avoid most cold cuts; high in fat)
Brazil nuts (unsalted)
cashews (unsalted)
cheese, all kinds (lean, low-fat such as edam best)
cheeses (lean or low-fat)
chicken, skinless
cottage cheese
crabmeat
cream cheese (low-fat is best)
dairy products of all kinds (look for low-fat)
eggs, (hard-boiled, scrambled, or omelet)
fish fillets of all kinds, baked or broiled
flounder
haddock
ham (lean only—no glaze)
hamburger (lean only)
lamb (lean)
lobster
meats, all kinds (lean is best; avoid high-fat cold cuts)
meat sauce over pasta
melon pieces
milk, skim or 2%
mozzarella, low-fat
nuts of all kinds
peanuts (unsalted; beware high calories)
pork tenderloin, well trimmed
ribs (lean, with light barbecue sauce okay)
salmon (baked, broiled, smoked)
sandwich, turkey or chicken on grain bread with lettuce, 1 tsp. mayo
sausage (lean)

scallops, sea
seafood, all kinds
   (avoid fried, sautéed)
seeds (pumpkin,
   sunflower, sesame)
shellfish, all kinds
shrimp (not fried)
sole
soybean products
   (beware of high
   calories)

steaks, beef all kinds
   (sirloin, T-bone . . .)
swordfish
tuna (packed in water)
turkey, skinned
veal (avoid sautéed)
walnuts (unsalted)
yogurt (low-fat or plain
   is best)

Second Best: High-Fiber, Low-Fat Carbohydrates

bran muffins
fruits, nonstarchy
apples
apricots (dried or
   fresh)
bananas
berries
melon
plums
raisins
fruit-and-nut mixtures,

such as trail mixes
   (low-salt)
**vegetables,
nonstarchy**
carrots (sticks)
celery (sticks, stuffed
   with cheese spread)
chickpeas (fresh,
   roasted)
cucumber (strips)
peppers, red or green
zucchini or summer
   squash

Sleep-Inducing Foods

High-Carbohydrate

These may contain protein ingredients, but in smaller proportion than carbohydrates. If eating a combination, eat carbohydrates first so that the brain releases serotonin. Items in bold are classes of foods; others are examples of snacks you may wish to carry in-flight or eat during a stopover.

apples, all forms
applesauce
apricots, all forms
bagels (with 2 tsp. jelly okay)
bananas
barley
beverages, sweetened
biscotti
bloody mary mix with celery sticks
bran flakes
bran muffins
breads, all kinds
breadsticks
cakes, all kinds
candy, all kinds (no chocolate)
cappuccino, decaffeinated
cereals, all kinds (no milk)
cereal, sugar-coated (no milk)
chips, all kinds
cookies, all kinds
corn, any kind
corn cakes, fat-free
cornbread or corn muffins
crackers, all kinds
cranberries
cranberry juice
crepes (no meat filling)
croissants, plain
diet supplement drinks (watch calories)

English muffin, plain
French toast with
    syrup
fig cookies
fruit cup, individual
fruit, dried rolls
ginger snaps
graham crackers
grains, all kinds
granola bar, low-fat
grapefruit
grapes
gumdrops
hard candy
honey
puddings, fat-free
    nonrefrigerated
ice cream, low-fat
jelly beans
juice (fruit)
Jujubes
muffins, all kinds (no
    butter, 1 tsp. jelly)
nectarines
noodles, all kinds
oatmeal
oranges
orange juice
pancakes (with syrup
    okay)
pasta, all kinds (avoid
    meat sauces)

pastry, all kinds
peaches
peanut butter (2 tbsp.
    with jelly in
    sandwich; cookies;
    crackers)
pies, all kinds
pickles
pineapples
pizza, all kinds
plums
popcorn, caramel-
    coated
popcorn, unbuttered
potatoes, all kinds
    (avoid fried,
    sautéed)
pretzels, low-salt
prunes
raisins
raspberries
rice
rice-marshmallow
    snacks
rice cakes
rolls, all kinds
soft drinks,
    sweetened
    (nondiet)
strawberries
sugar, all kinds

sweet potato
tacos, all
tortillas
tangerines

vegetables, most
watermelon
wheat cereal
wheat bread

Sources: Jean Carper, *Food: Your Miracle Medicine;* Judith Wurtman, *Managing Your Mind and Mood through Food;* Art Ulene, M.D., *Book of Food Counts.*

Source Directory for Jet Lag Tools

Diets

The Anti–Jet Lag Diet
Argonne National Laboratory
9700 South Cass Ave.
Argonne, IL 60439

Send stamped, self-addressed envelope to receive wallet-size overview card of Charles F. Ehret's anti–jet lag diet.

Managing Your Mind and Mood through Food
by Judith J. Wurtman, Ph.D.

More details and techniques from prominent research scientist explaining interaction of carbohydrates and proteins and how to use the knowledge to help reset your body clocks.

Light Therapy Devices

MedEd Publications
PO Box 12415
Columbus, OH 43212
 Write for their consumer's guide to light therapy devices.

Many companies now manufacture and sell artificial 10,000 lux light devices, including floor-model and portable light boxes (many portable suitable for travel), lighted visors, or dawn-to-sundown-simulating lighting devices. A few are listed here:

Apollo Light Systems, Inc.
352 West 1060 St.
South Orem, UT 84058
800-545-9667
801-226-2370
 Floor model and portable light boxes; dawn-simulating alarm clock.

Bio-Brite, Inc.
7315 Wisconsin Ave., 1300W
Bethesda, MD 20814-3202
800-621-LITE (5483)
 Company associated with NIMH doctor-author-researchers, which offered one of the first battery-operated headlight visors, now up-

dated; also portable light boxes and other products to relieve jet lag. A kit, to buy or rent, contains dark wraparound glasses, visor, cardboard trip calculator. (Also produces the lighted globe alarm clock noted in this book that slowly starts to shine thirty minutes before your alarm time, gradually illuminating room until alarm goes off.)

Environmental Lighting Concepts
3923 Coconut Palm Dr., Suite 101
Tampa, FL 33619
800-842-8848
813-621-0058
  Light boxes.

Health Light, Inc.
PO Box 3899
Station C
Hamilton, ON Canada L8H 7P2
1-800-265-6020
  Manufacturers of the Red Light Cap and a newer unit, Thera Clip, that clips into a pair of glasses, onto a cap or visor.

Lighting Resources
1421 W. Third Ave.
Columbus, OH 43212-2928
800-875-8489
614-488-6841
  A variety of permanent and portable light boxes; light visor.

Medic-Lite, Inc.
Yacht Club Dr.

Lake Hopatcong, NJ 07849
800-544-4825
   Light boxes; portable, head-mounted light visor.

Northern Light Technologies
PO Box 1801
Homer, AL 99603
1-800-880-6953
nlights@xyz.net
   Floor-model light box, plus compact adjustable
   unit.

Photon Therapeutics
26263 Via Roble
Mission Viejo, CA 92691-2568
714-951-7945
   Jet lag visor.

Pi Square, Inc.
11036 First Ave. S.
Seattle, WA 98168
800-786-3296
206-246-1101
   Portable and floor-model 10,000 lux light boxes,
   dawn-to-dusk simulator.

The SunBox Company
19217 Orbit Dr., Dept. PT
Gaithersburg, MD 20879
301-762-1786
800-548-3968
Floor-model and portable light boxes, light visor.

Wraparound Disposable Glasses

Wraparound sunglasses are now widely available commercially at drugstores. Disposable ones can be found.

Tecfen Corporation
5860-C Hollister Ave.
Santa Barbara, CA 93117
805-967-1153
tecfen@tecfen.com
  Manufacturers of SolarShield products.

Solarettes
Dioptics Medical Products
San Luis Obispo, CA 93401
  Solarettes are dark glasses that fit under regular dark glasses to provide more darkening.

Anti–Jet Lag Scheduling

How to Beat Jet Lag by Dan. A. Oren, M.D., Walter Reich, M.D., Norman E. Rosenthal, M.D., and Thomas A. Wehr, M.D.
  Paperback with charts and instructions for critical times of each flight, according to total time zones crossed, east and west. Package includes opaque eye mask, disposable wraparound dark glasses.

JET-READY Travel Services
Att.: Stop Jet Lag Recommendations
12672 Skyline Blvd.
Woodside, CA 94062
1-415-851-2457

Anti–jet lag diet author Charles Ehret uses his patented software to provide diet and light strategy for your specific trip itinerary. Contact eleven or more days prior to trip for lower price.

Index